W0232924

THE LITTLE BOOK OF IKIGAI

JO PETERS

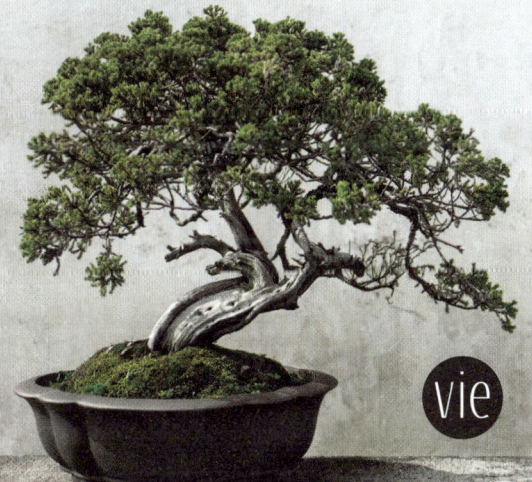

vie

THE LITTLE BOOK OF IKIGAI

Copyright © Octopus Publishing Group Limited, 2025

All rights reserved.

Text by Emily Kearns

No part of this book may be reproduced by any means, nor transmitted, nor translated into a machine language, without the written permission of the publishers.

Condition of Sale
This book is sold subject to the condition that it shall not, by way of trade or otherwise, be lent, resold, hired out or otherwise circulated in any form of binding or cover other than that in which it is published and without a similar condition including this condition being imposed on the subsequent purchaser.

An Hachette UK Company
www.hachette.co.uk

Vie Books, an imprint of Summersdale Publishers
Part of Octopus Publishing Group Limited
Carmelite House
50 Victoria Embankment
LONDON
EC4Y 0DZ
UK

www.summersdale.com

This FSC® label means that materials and other controlled sources used for the product have been responsibly sourced

MIX
Paper | Supporting responsible forestry
FSC® C018236

The authorized representative in the EEA is Hachette Ireland, 8 Castlecourt Centre, Dublin 15, D15 XTP3, Ireland (email: info@hbgi.ie)

Printed and bound in Poland

ISBN: 978-1-83799-717-6
eISBN: 978-1-83799-718-3

Substantial discounts on bulk quantities of Summersdale books are available to corporations, professional associations and other organizations. For details contact general enquiries: telephone: +44 (0) 1243 771107 or email: enquiries@summersdale.com.

CONTENTS

INTRODUCTION

You might be familiar with the term "ikigai", or it might be completely new to you. For the uninitiated, ikigai is quite simply your reason for being, your *raison d'être*, but with many layers. "Ikigai" itself is a blending of two Japanese words: "iki" meaning "life" and "gai" meaning "reason". This Japanese philosophy is ultimately about finding balance and purpose in your life by focusing on the things you enjoy. Many claim its teachings hold the secrets to a long, happy and meaningful existence.

The concept of ikigai originated in the Okinawa Islands more than a thousand years ago and was adopted into Japanese culture in the years that followed. In more recent times, the idea of ikigai has spread to the West, where devotees harness its teachings to find meaning in their day-to-day lives.

The key to ikigai lies in dedication and patience. It invites you to embark on a journey of self-discovery to find your true passion, mission, vocation and profession – the four elements of ikigai. These four elements fall into categories known as the four pillars of ikigai: what you love, what the world needs, what you are good at and what you can be paid for.

The Japanese believe that everyone has an ikigai just waiting to be discovered. Some people unlock theirs with relative ease, while others spend years searching for it.

This book will take you on a journey through the history, philosophy and cultural significance of ikigai, stopping to look at the four pillars in greater detail, before offering ways in which you can discover your ikigai and use it to find meaning in your life. Along the way, you'll be introduced to other Japanese life concepts and discover how these fit into the bigger picture and, crucially, how they relate to ikigai.

Perhaps most importantly, in these pages you will learn how to incorporate ikigai into your life and how, through regular practice, you can sustain it, reaping the benefits of the balance and fulfilment it can bring. Here you will find a range of daily practices, from journalling to self-reflection and visualization, as well as advice on how to calm your mind to help you find and maintain your ikigai and useful tips on hobbies, goal setting and career moves.

Your ikigai is a part of you just waiting to be discovered. So, what are you waiting for?

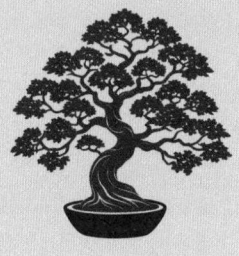

THE
ORIGINS
OF
IKIGAI

This chapter explains the origins of ikigai and how it fits into modern life, as well as touching on other Japanese life concepts and how they slot into the bigger picture. While the practice of ikigai has been embedded in Japanese culture for centuries, its origins can be traced back to a place in Japan called Okinawa, where the sense of ikigai remains particularly strong to this day – you could even say it is stronger here than anywhere else in the world.

Okinawa is known for its close-knit community and unusually high number of 100-year-olds. Alongside particular diet and lifestyle choices, the drive to pursue their ikigai well into their golden years is thought to be key to residents' longevity.

This chapter is your chance to unlock the benefits of an ancient philosophy that could shift your perspective and bring joy and purpose to your life.

WHERE IT ALL BEGAN

While the word "ikigai" can be traced back in Japanese history to the Heian period (794–1185), the birthplace of the concept of ikigai is to be found in the prefecture of Okinawa, an archipelago of more than 150 islands in the East China Sea, where many inhabitants enjoy a long existence thought to be due to their life choices. Okinawans put their longevity down to the adoption of ikigai as a way of life and believe that in seeking purpose through this philosophy they have found health, happiness and fulfilment.

Island residents are said to suffer from some of the lowest levels of dementia, cancer and heart disease in the world, which they attribute to the fact that they have worked to find meaning in their existence and learned the art of balance in all areas of their lives. Okinawans describe ikigai as their reason for getting up in the morning and many find their purpose for being through working or keeping up with hobbies well into old age. (See page 19 for the Okinawans' "ten rules of ikigai".)

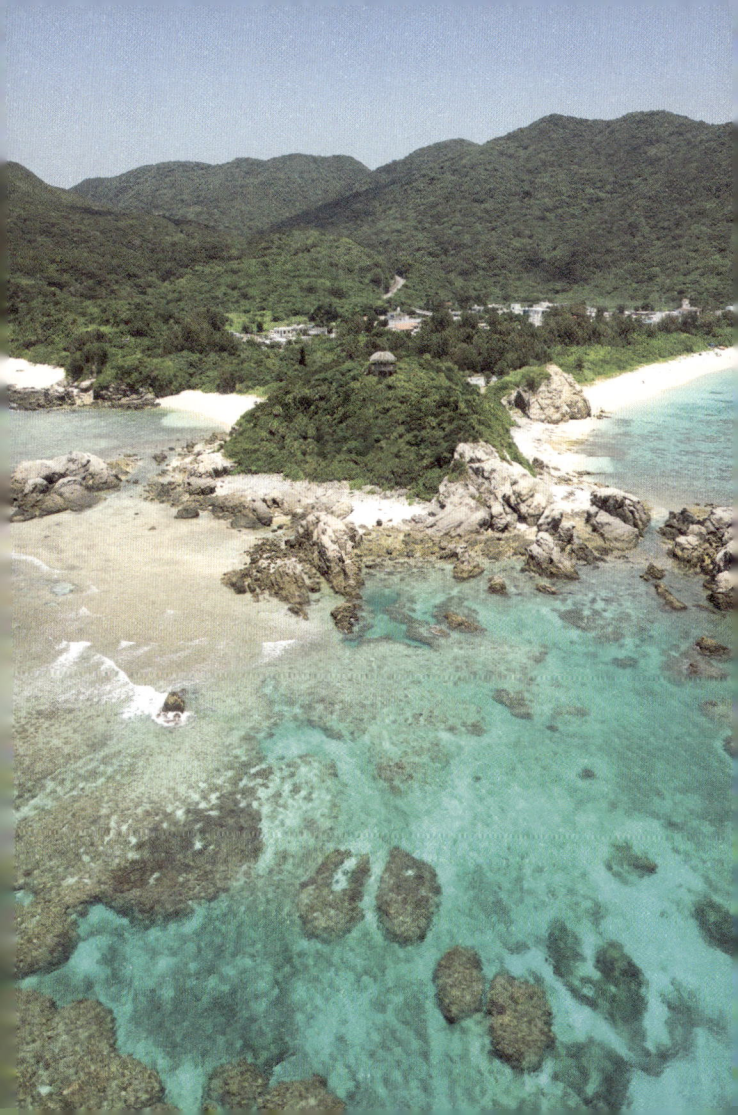

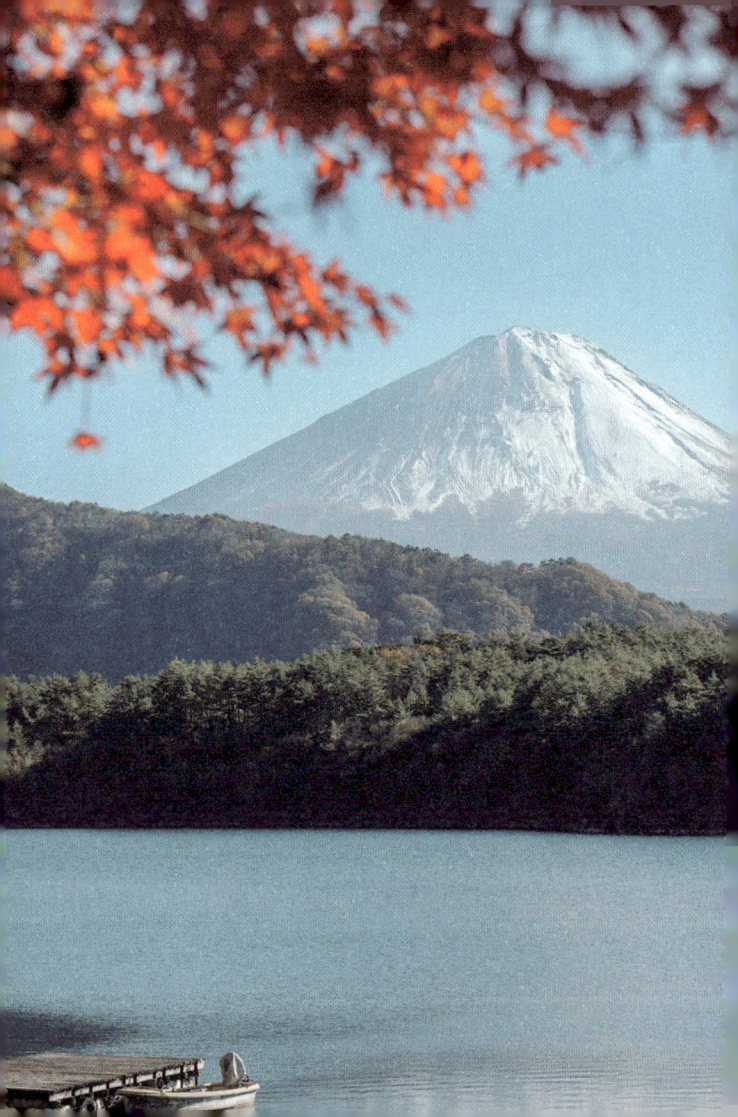

CULTURAL SIGNIFICANCE

While the specific meaning of ikigai in Japanese culture and beyond is explored in these pages, it is important to remember that the word is part of a wider cultural tradition in Japan, which is a country well known for its many life philosophies. These concepts are often encapsulated in a single word that open us up to a new way of viewing the world (see page 12 for examples). Ikigai is just one of these philosophies and in fact the word is so commonplace in Japan that it is often used casually, with "feeling a sense of ikigai" interchangeable with "feeling alive".

As with many of these concepts, ikigai is something that people naturally lean towards in Japan, ingrained as it is in the way of life. Experts are keen to stress that a person's ikigai evolves throughout the course of their life. It is a multifaceted concept that grows with us – we may discover more than just one true purpose over our lifetime.

JAPANESE LIFE CONCEPTS

As we have seen, ikigai is just one of many Japanese life philosophies we can all learn from and adopt. Below are some of the others.

- **Wabi-sabi** – This idea encourages us to admire imperfection and find beauty in transience. It follows three basic tenets: nothing lasts, nothing is finished and nothing is perfect.

- **Oubaitori** – This is about never comparing yourself to others. The word "oubaitori" comes from the kanji for the apricot, cherry, plum and peach trees that bloom in spring. Ultimately, the message is that everyone blossoms in their own way and at their own pace.

- **Mottainai** – This is the idea that everything on the planet deserves respect and therefore we should not be wasteful. By following this philosophy, you should work to respect the value of resources and, if you don't already, champion the notion of reducing, reusing and recycling.

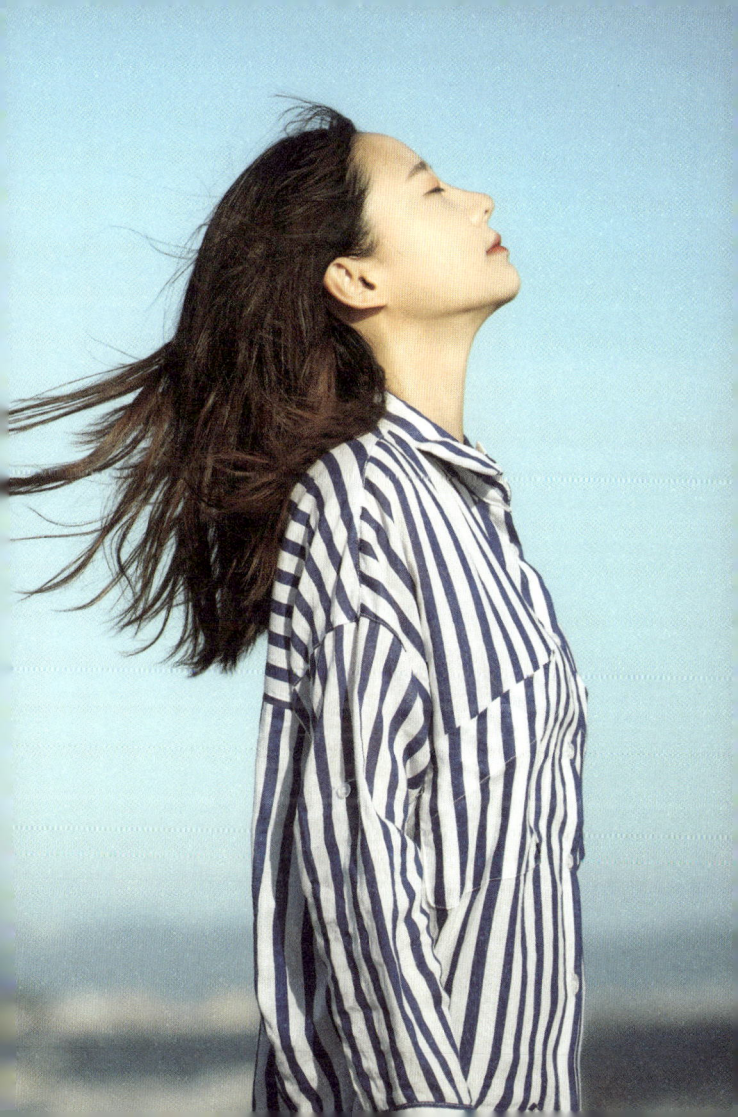

*I took a walk in the woods and
came out taller than the trees.*

HENRY DAVID THOREAU

JAPANESE LIFE
CONCEPTS AND IKIGAI

Many Japanese philosophies place emphasis on kindness and gratitude, promote self-improvement and encourage a more mindful existence, all of which can be useful in the search for ikigai.

For example, *kaizen* is the idea that if you are always improving in all areas of your life, you are constantly fine-tuning the effectiveness of everything you choose to do. This perpetual improvement can be gentle and gradual, reminding us of the importance of maintaining momentum.

Shinrin-yoku, or "forest bathing", meanwhile, is about spending time immersed in the natural world, accepting and acknowledging the present moment and allowing nature to both heal and benefit your health.

THE POPULARIZATION
OF IKIGAI

While the concept of ikigai is centuries old, it was brought into the Japanese mainstream in 1966 by the book *Ikigai ni Tsuite* ("About Ikigai") by psychiatrist and translator Mieko Kamiya and published in the West under the title *On the Meaning of Life*. Kamiya believed that when someone experiences ikigai at its fullest, this gives them a personal mission in life.

In more recent years, ikigai has been pushed further into the global spotlight thanks to the publication in 2016 of *Ikigai: The Japanese Secret to a Long and Happy Life* by Héctor García and Francesc Miralles. The pair interviewed more than a hundred Okinawans from Ogimi – often referred to as "the village of longevity" – and discovered that every one of them had an ikigai. Recognizing that ikigai is for the young as well as the old, in 2021 García and Miralles published *Ikigai for Teens: Finding Your Reason for Being*.

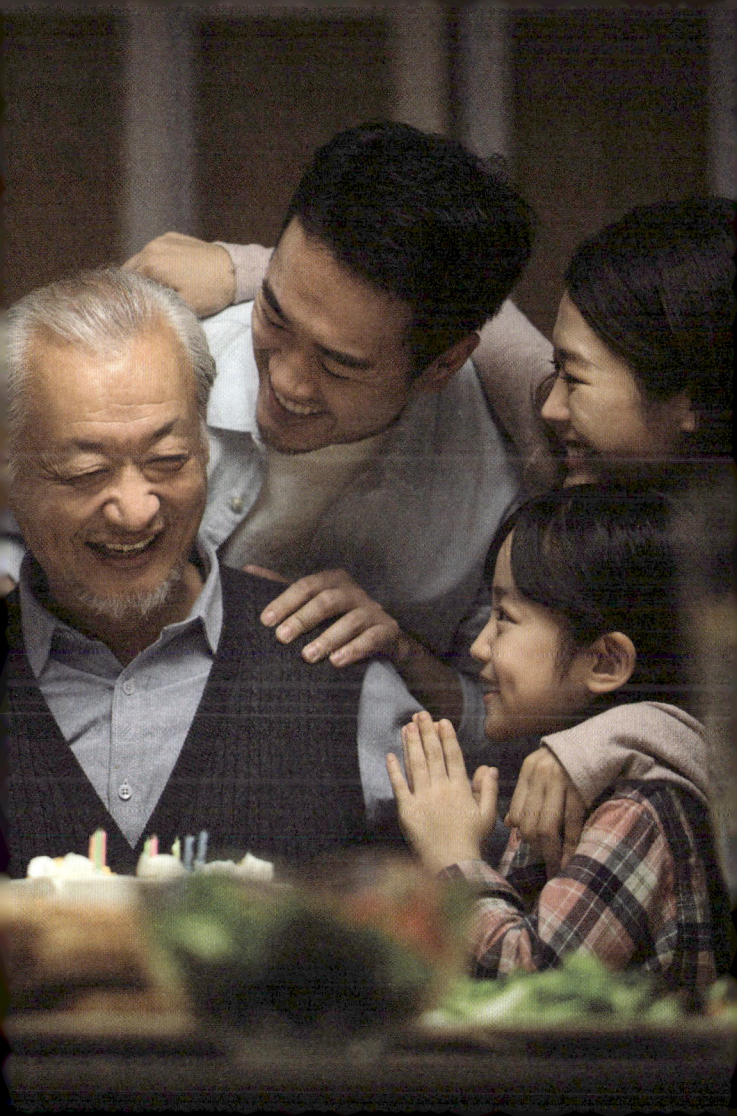

 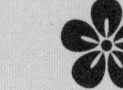

TO AGE WELL
IS TO EMBRACE
CHANGE AND
ENJOY LIFE'S
EVOLUTION

THE TEN RULES OF IKIGAI

In their book *Ikigai: The Japanese Secret to a Long and Happy Life*, García and Miralles looked to the centenarians of Okinawa to impart their wisdom and share their secret to longevity. The following ideas were deemed by the Okinawans to be integral to their long and fulfilled life and these have been widely adopted in the West as a framework for ikigai:

1.   Stay active. Don't retire.
2.   Take it slow.
3.   Don't fill your stomach.
4.   Surround yourself with good friends.
5.   Get in shape for your next birthday.
6.   Smile.
7.   Reconnect with nature.
8.   Give thanks.
9.   Live in the moment.
10. Follow your ikigai.

IKIGAI IN MODERN TIMES

The *Oxford English Dictionary* describes ikigai as "a motivating force" that "gives a person a sense of purpose or a reason for living". In the modern world, you might find your ikigai through exploration of your talents, whether at work or play, or in helping others; you might find it within your family, by heading outdoors, or through exercise, yoga or meditation. Mindful activities, and pausing to reflect – along with creating a sense of space and time to consider your thoughts – are all useful in the search for your ikigai.

It all boils down to finding enjoyment in life through each of the four pillars – what you love (your passion – this could be family or a hobby), what the world needs (your mission – perhaps volunteering, raising money for a charitable cause or working towards change for good), what you are good at (your vocation – where your talents lie) and what you can be paid for (your profession).

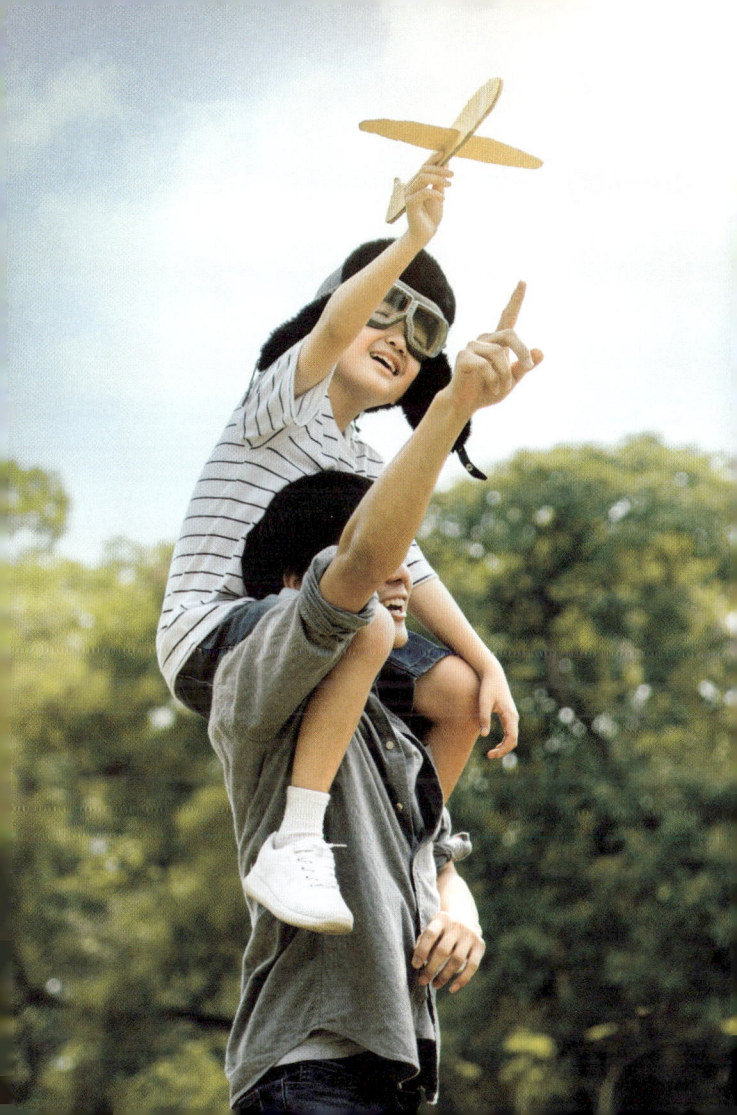

IKIGAI AND WELL-BEING IN THE WEST

With mental health brought more into focus in recent years, many argue that ikigai should be part of the healthcare process in the West in helping those with depression seek purpose and reasons to get up in the morning.

In 2019, Dr Dean Fido and Yasuhiro Kotera at the University of Derby collaborated with Kenichi Asano in Japan to carry out a UK research project to measure the impacts of ikigai on a sample of 349 participants (with an average age of 35).

The aim was to discover the effects of the pursuit of ikigai on participants alongside "previously established and validated measures of well-being, depression, anxiety and stress". The study found that the greater the presence of ikigai reported by participants, the better their well-being and, crucially, the lower their symptoms of depression.

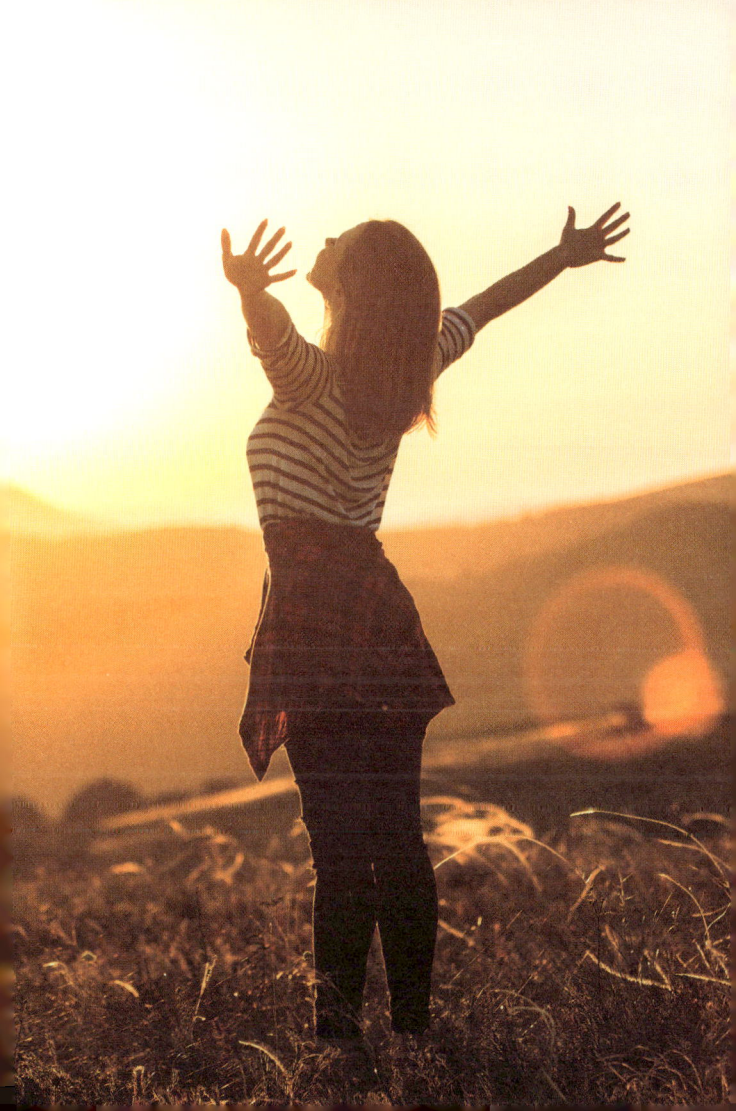

INTERPRETATIONS OF IKIGAI

In the West, ikigai is represented by a Venn diagram that sees the four pillars overlapping to guide you towards finding a sense of purpose – your ikigai. This Venn diagram was adopted as a means to express the Japanese life concept in an easily digestible and approachable way (see page 34). However, it's worth bearing in mind that purists such as Ken Mogi, who was raised in Japan and was immersed in the concept from a young age, believe the philosophy can be practised and achieved without all four pillars being addressed. Mogi holds that ikigai doesn't need to be approached in "rule-based algorithmic ways" and instead his interpretation looks to five pillars:

1. Starting small
2. Releasing yourself
3. Harmony and sustainability
4. The joy of little things
5. Being in the here and now

While Mogi's ideas are in a more organic form, this book will use the structured Venn diagram approach to help you on your ikigai journey.

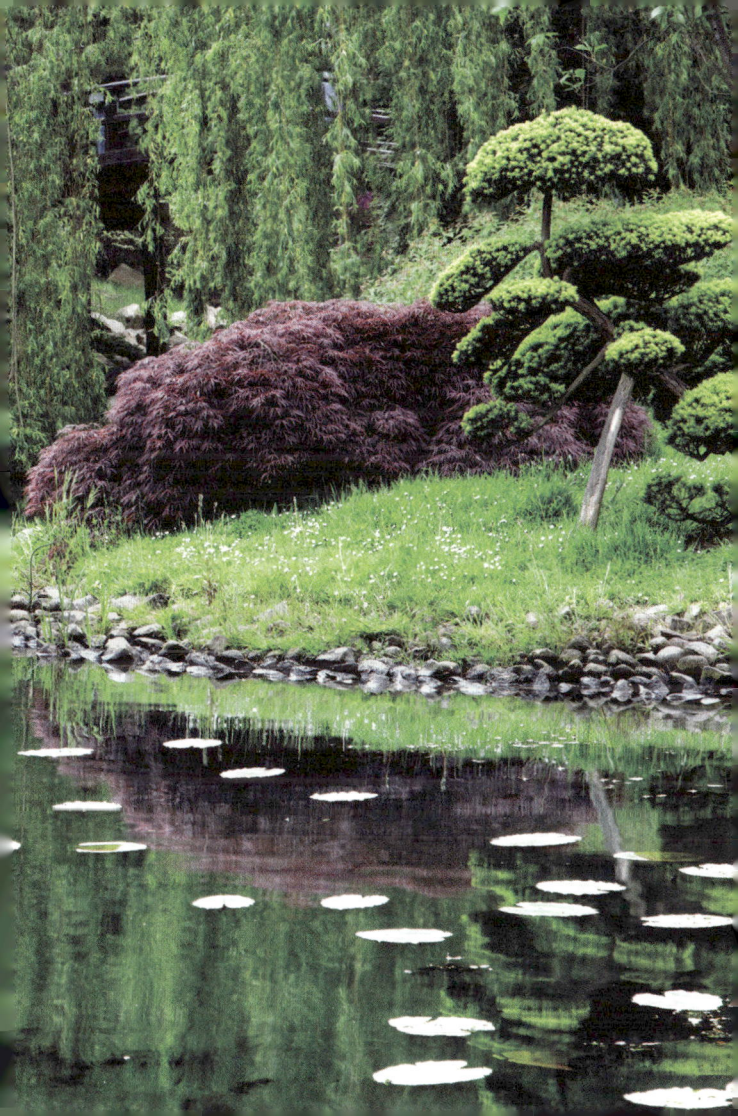

*Ikigai is the action we take
in pursuit of happiness.*

YUKARI MITSUHASHI

WORDS OF WISDOM

So, what makes for a long and healthy life? According to Polish-American chemist Dr Alexander Imich, who lived to be 111, a healthy diet, alcohol abstention, exercise, meditation and nutritional supplements are key; while Japanese woman Kane Tanaka, who lived to be 119, claimed her large family, positivity, hope, good food, an early morning routine and practising maths was what kept her alive for so long.

What do you think might keep you going into old age? Consider Imich and Tanaka's responses and how they cover purpose, lifestyle and enjoyment – all key areas to unlocking your ikigai. Take a pen and paper and write down what you think you might say if asked the same question as Imich and Tanaka at the age of 100. Your responses will be useful as you make your way through this book and progress towards your own ikigai.

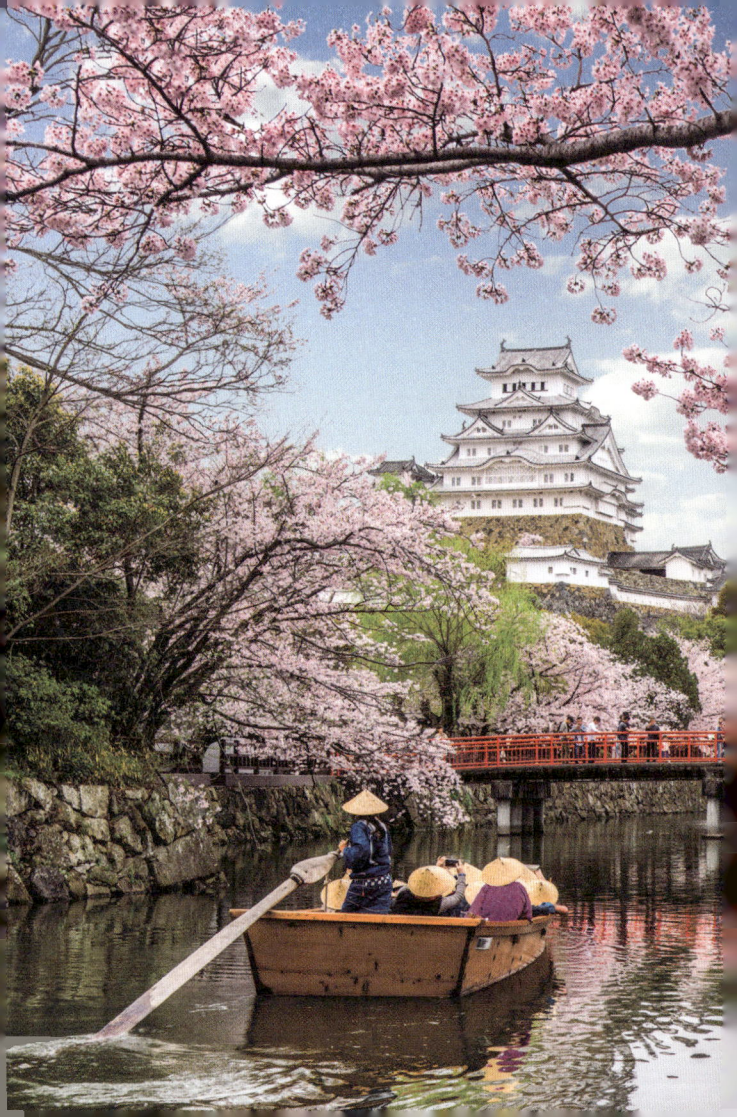

KEY IKIGAI FIGURES

These people have been instrumental in bringing ikigai to the masses:

- **Héctor García and Francesc Miralles** – Co-authors of 2016's *Ikigai: The Japanese Secret to a Long and Happy Life*, the pair are responsible for the take-up of ikigai on a global scale, particularly in the West.

- **Mieko Kamiya** – Kamiya is the author of the seminal 1966 book *Ikigai ni Tsuite (On the Meaning of Life)* and is responsible for popularizing ikigai in modern times. Often referred to as the "mother of ikigai", psychiatrist Kamiya paved the way for the movement and famously found her own ikigai in her writing.

- **Tim Tamashiro** – Calling himself the "ikigai guy", Tamashiro is a motivational speaker on all things ikigai and author of several books including *How to Ikigai* and *Ikigai: Do What You Love*. He has given TED Talks about ikigai and refers to the philosophy as a map and the four pillars as the directions.

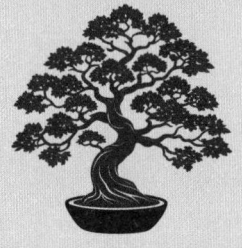

THE
FOUR
PILLARS

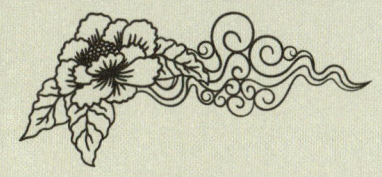

The four pillars are the essential areas you should focus on when it comes to unlocking your ikigai. These are key to seeking your purpose and fulfilment. As we have seen, the four pillars are what you love (passion), what the world needs (mission), what you are good at (vocation) and what you can be paid for (profession).

This chapter looks at each of these areas in more detail to help you on your journey and introduces you to the ikigai Venn diagram, which will enlighten you as to where the pillars overlap and help you make sense of it all.

This understanding marks the next phase of your journey to finding enjoyment and satisfaction in your life. So, are you ready to take the next step on your path to purpose? Read on to learn more about the pillars and how these can inform your ikigai.

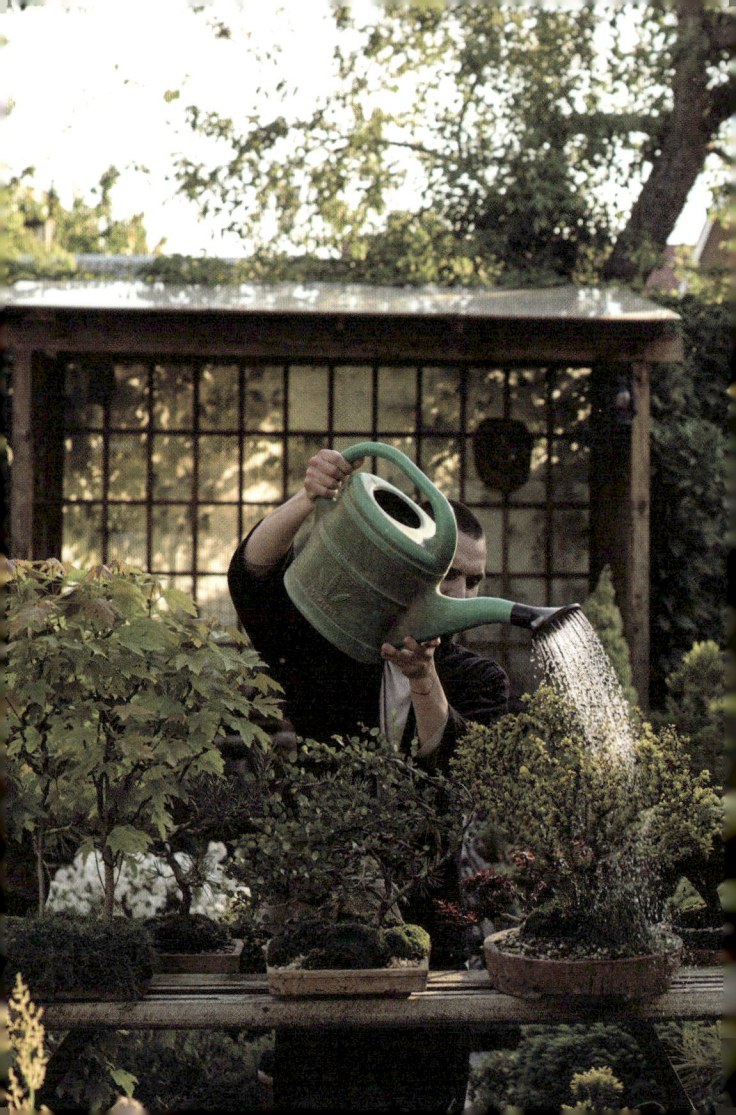

THE FOUR PILLARS OF IKIGAI

- **What you love** – These are the activities that you enjoy so much that you become absorbed in them and often lose track of time. Perhaps you feel this way about a hobby or maybe it's spending time with people you love.

- **What the world needs** – These are the things you see the world needs help with. What can you do to make it a better place? It doesn't matter how small; you can still make a change.

- **What you are good at** – These are your skills and natural talents. Perhaps you are good at public speaking or have baking down to a fine art. You might be a particularly good listener or problem-solver, or maybe you excel at sports.

- **What you can be paid for** – This is your employed work; the job that earns you money. In an ideal world your job reflects the other three pillars.

THE IKIGAI VENN DIAGRAM

Look at the diagram on the next page. You can see how the elements of ikigai come together. Where the circles (pillars) overlap, so do the elements:

- **Passion** = What you love and what you are good at
- **Mission** = What you love and what the world needs
- **Vocation** = What the world needs and what you can be paid for
- **Profession** = What you are good at and what you can be paid for

Finding something you love that you are good at, something the world needs that you love, something you can be paid for that the world needs and something you're good at that you can be paid for are all part of the process. While this formula is widely used in the search for ikigai, some feel it deviates somewhat from the original meaning of the concept (see page 38); the Venn diagram suggests a destination, but the ancient practice is very much about the journey.

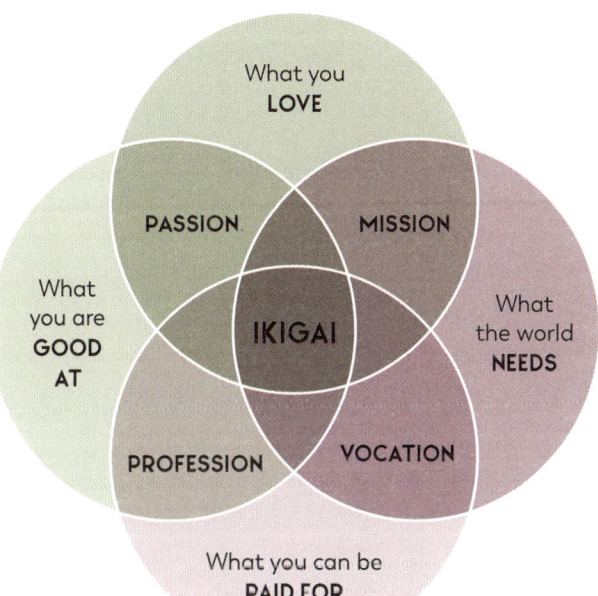

What you LOVE

What the world NEEDS

What you can be PAID FOR

What you are GOOD AT

PASSION

MISSION

IKIGAI

PROFESSION

VOCATION

THE INTERSECTION OF THE VENN DIAGRAM

Look at the Venn diagram on page 35. You'll see a middle space where all four pillars overlap. *This* is where you will find your ikigai. It is here where you will find the balance between the four pillars, and, in aligning the stages of your journey (to encompass your passion, mission, vocation and profession), you find a sense of purpose. This middle spot is the ultimate goal and the pillars are integral to finding your ikigai. If you can focus on these four vital life areas, you'll be on your way.

Notice that there are four segments in the Venn diagram where three of the circles (pillars) overlap. It might sound appealing and more achievable to combine three rather than all four – reaching these places *will* bring a sense of satisfaction and happiness – but you will always be lacking the crucial benefits of the missing pillar.

*The prime of your life
does not come twice.*

JAPANESE PROVERB

THE HISTORY OF THE IKIGAI VENN DIAGRAM

The Venn diagram associated with ikigai stems from the "Venn diagram of purpose" created by Spanish astrologer Andrés Zuzunaga in 2011. Zuzunaga confessed to the Ikigai Tribe podcast in 2021 that he knew little about the Japanese life concept and did not have it in mind when he put the diagram together.

In 2014, business coach and entrepreneur Marc Winn wrote a blog post about ikigai in which he merged the Venn diagram of purpose with his interpretation of ikigai. The blog post went viral and the diagram has been widely adopted as a template for ikigai and it has come to represent the concept in the Western world.

Ikigai purists, such as Ken Mogi (see page 24), view this Venn diagram with some suspicion, but Winn argues it has unintentionally transformed the lives of millions of people who have gone on to discover their ikigai and therefore their purpose in life.

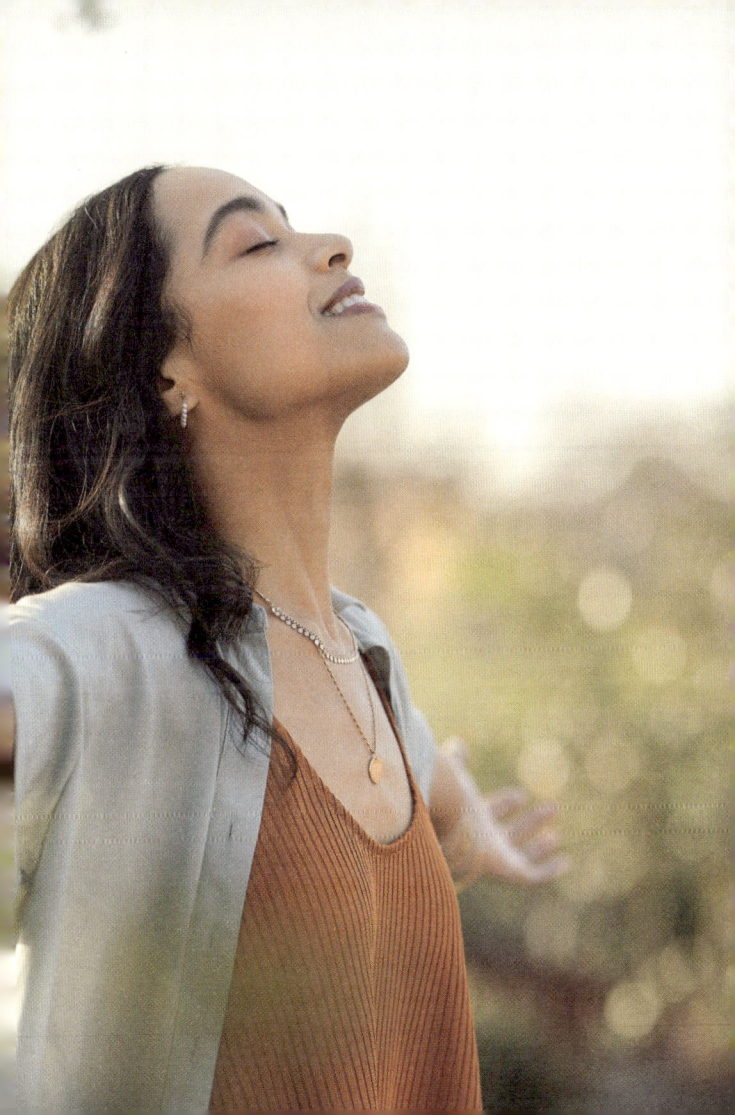

DOING WHAT YOU LOVE: PASSION/MISSION

This aspect of ikigai sees two of the four elements overlap under the first pillar – doing what you love. This pillar is all about seeking out the things in life that bring you joy. These joyful activities should be ones that you can lose yourself in; you are so immersed in what you are doing that you lose track of time and achieve a state of "flow".

Your joyful activity might be creative, such as painting, crocheting or writing; you might lose yourself in music, dancing, or both; or perhaps your green-fingered soul is happiest planting and weeding in the garden. Spending time with pets, family members or friends who know you better than anyone might be where your joy lies; or perhaps it's cooking, reading, walking in nature or running along the coast. Ikigai teaches us that incorporating joyful activities into our lives is essential for achieving a good balance of happiness and well-being.

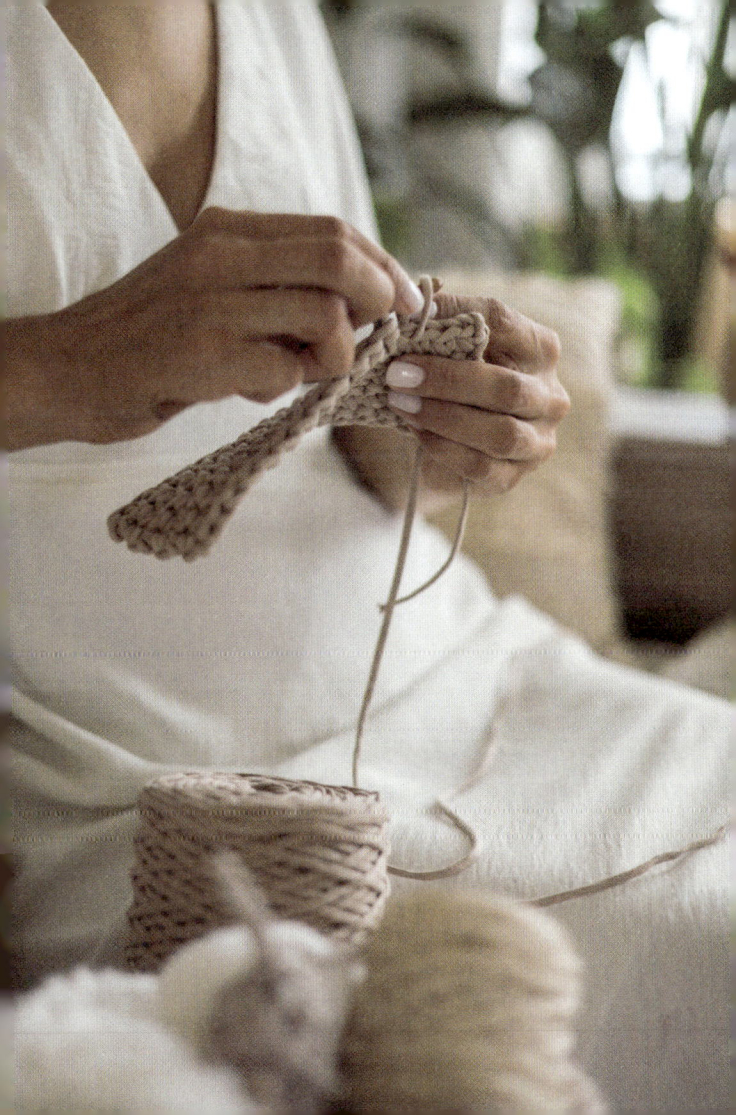

SEEKING YOUR PASSION

While some people find themselves easily drawn to activities and leisure pursuits that interest them and provide joy, others find it more difficult to identify and seek these out. If this is the case for you, approaching hobbies and interests with an open mind is likely to pay off. Speak to friends and family – the people who know you best – about what they feel might be right for you and take the time to consider things you may have dismissed in the past.

As we go through different stages of life, our needs and desires develop and evolve, so something that wasn't right a few years ago might bring you fulfilment now. As well as bringing essential health benefits, no matter how solitary your activity, there will always be a community of like-minded others for you to connect with.

HAPPY ARE
THOSE WHO
HAVE FOUND
THEIR PURPOSE

WHAT THE WORLD NEEDS: MISSION/VOCATION

This aspect of ikigai sees two of the four elements overlap under the second pillar – what the world needs. This is all about working out how you can help others and make change. This could be at a grass-roots level within your community, such as volunteering your time and resources to make a difference. Or you might have the capacity to effect greater change at a national or organizational level, perhaps through connections, knowledge or talent.

Ask yourself what the world needs and how you could help – even in some small way – to bring about a greater good. Consider how you would like others to remember you – putting the needs of others first is a great stepping stone on the path to finding your ikigai.

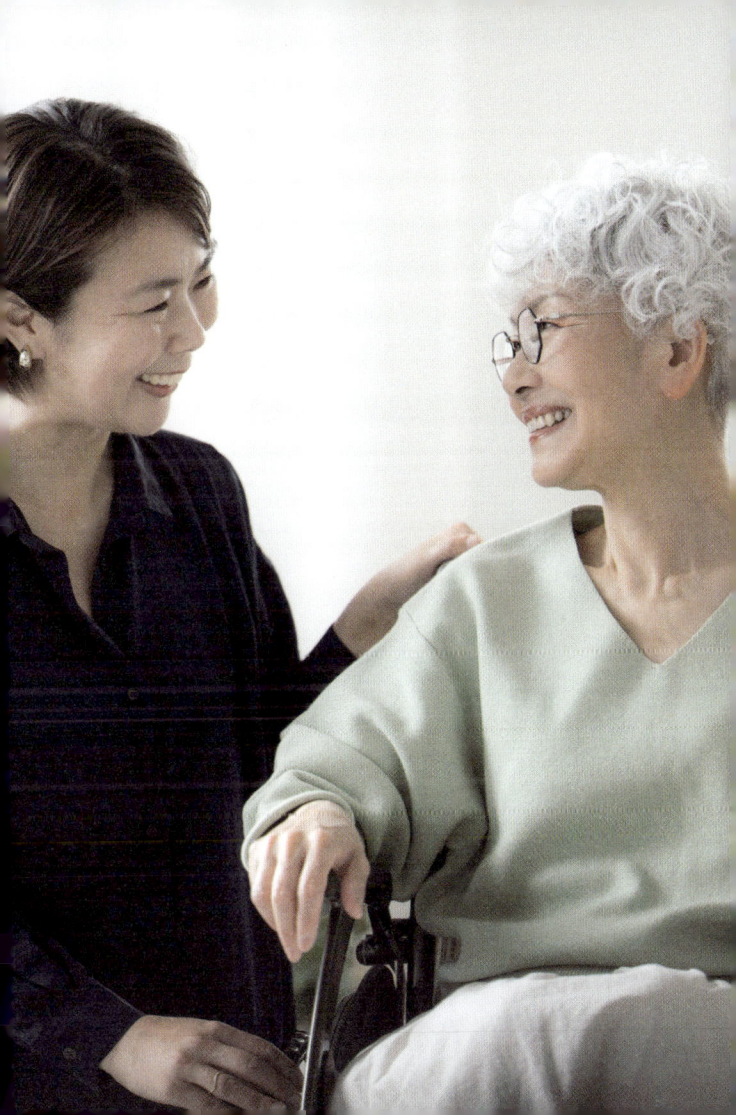

ENSURE YOUR LIFE IS A MISSION, RATHER THAN AN INTERMISSION

There is no greater love than
to give humans their ikigai.

MIEKO KAMIYA

WHAT YOU ARE GOOD AT: PASSION/PROFESSION

This aspect of ikigai sees two of the four elements overlap under the third pillar – what you are good at. This might be one you can answer quite easily, but there's much to consider in order to achieve the overlap between passion and profession.

Think about where your strengths lie in terms of what you like to do in your personal time – what have your achievements been throughout your life? What comes easily to you? Perhaps you are skilled in a particular area or have a natural flair for something. Whatever it is, pursue it. It could be the key to unlocking the ikigai puzzle. It's also important to think about what success means to you when working towards combining your passion and your profession.

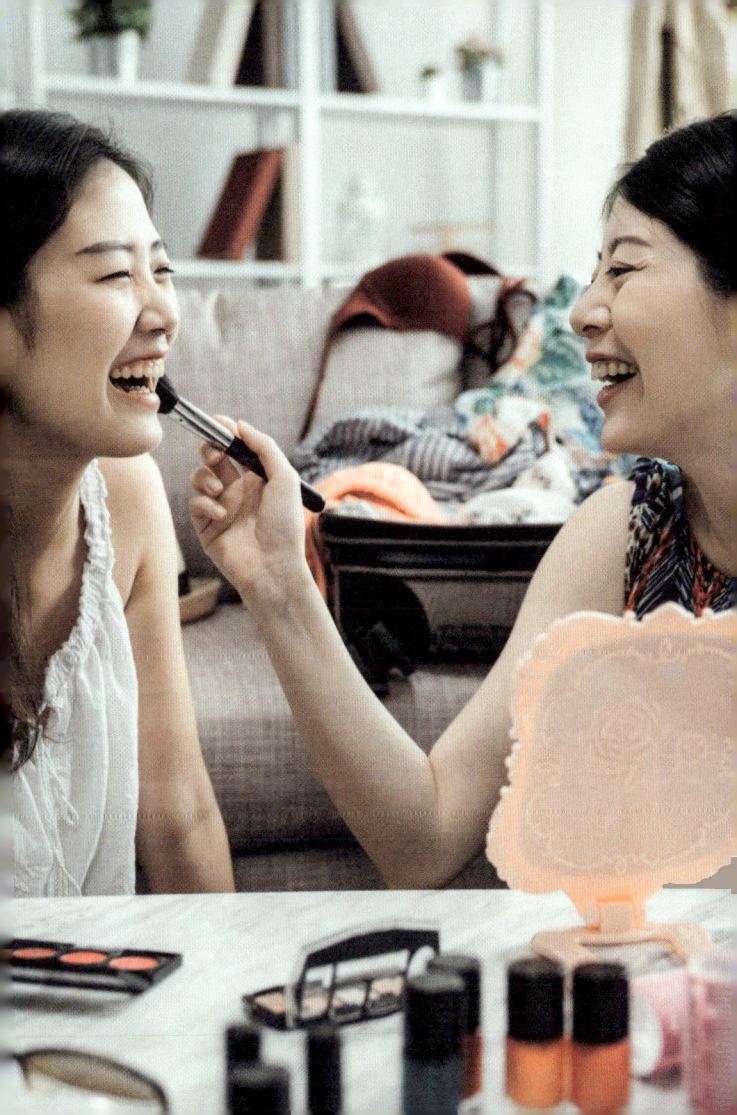

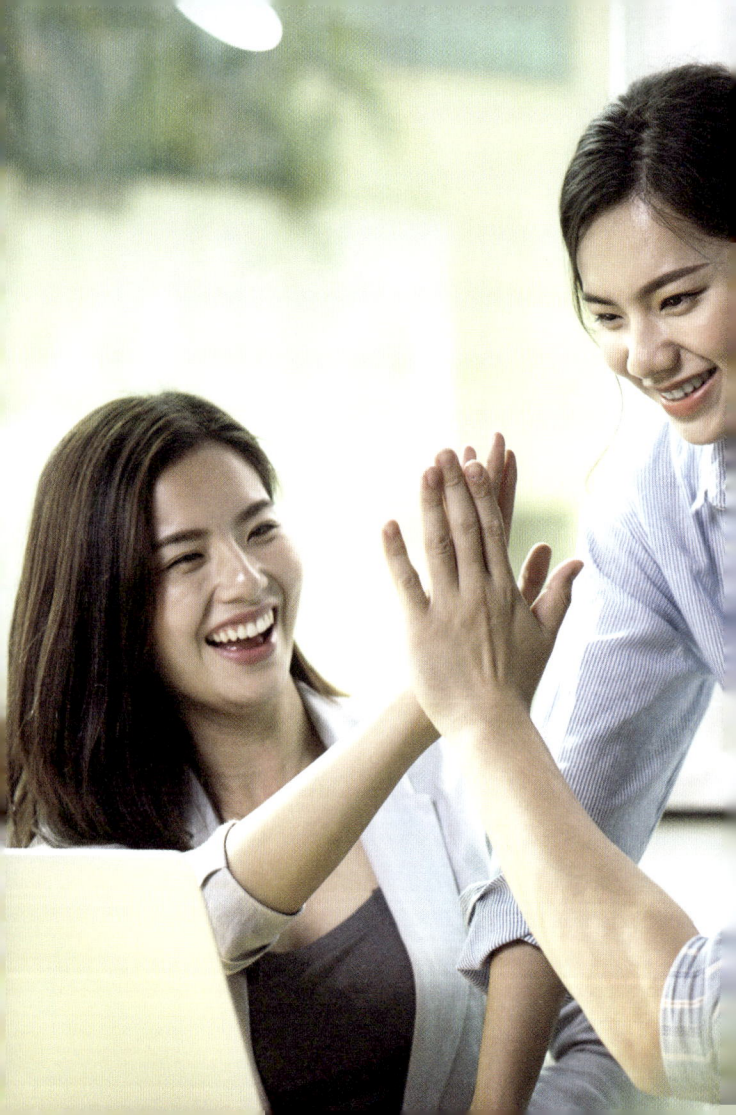

WHAT YOU CAN BE PAID FOR: PROFESSION/VOCATION

This aspect of ikigai sees two of the four elements overlap under the fourth pillar – what you can be paid for. While the type of job you do is important, you also want to consider the environment in which you work, as well as the hours and terms. All of these components will contribute to your well-being, financially, physically and emotionally.

Consider how much you need to earn to cover your expenses. Do you want to earn more, or could you potentially earn less and enjoy more time to pursue leisure activities or do volunteering work (what you love and what the world needs)? Think about where your skills lie and where they could naturally thrive, as well as what you enjoy, who you would be willing to work for and the values that are important to you.

IKIGAI DOS AND DON'TS

DO

- Consider why you do things
- Try something new
- Take time to make decisions
- Focus on the positive impact you can have on your community
- Try to form new habits for the better

DON'T

- Be worried about standing out
- Be dismissive if you don't take to something straight away
- Rush into things
- Try to save the world
- Beat yourself up if you miss a day or can't stick to it; you can always try again

CHOOSE A
JOB YOU LOVE,
AND YOU WILL
THANK YOURSELF
EVERY DAY

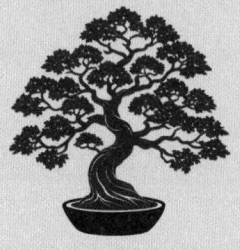

DISCOVERING YOUR IKIGAI

Finding the balance between the four pillars to achieve fulfilment across all areas of your life is a goal worth striving for. Seeking satisfaction in life involves embarking on a search within yourself. So it can be helpful to make time for reflection, rather than diving in head-first, and the following pages will help you with this. By reframing how you approach disparate areas of your life as you reach for your ikigai, you will begin to view things in a different way.

This chapter offers a range of simple activities and practices that will not only help you work towards a healthy mind and body but give you the headspace you need to think about each of the four pillars, and how to make life changes in your quest for purpose.

BUILDING A DAILY PRACTICE

The first step on your ikigai journey involves creating some mental breathing space to find clarity and bring the four pillars together. Building a daily practice can really help clear your mind and pave the way for constructive thought. Whether you choose to commit to daily exercise, meditation, journalling or yoga, starting off small is key and will help you build up to something bigger to effect long-term change. Just 5–10 minutes each day is a good place to start, gently adding 30 seconds or a minute, every day or so.

The Japanese practice of *shukanka* (forming a new habit) comes into play here and is about making subtle changes you gradually build upon to alter your life path in the long term.

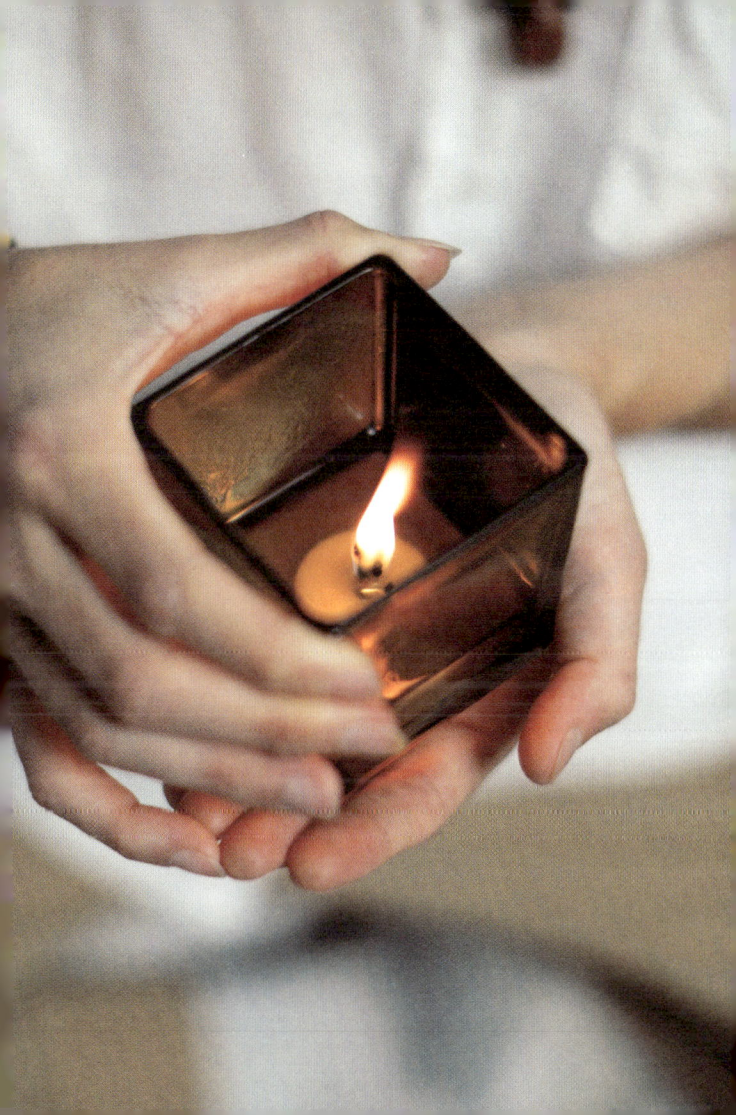

POSITIVE VS
NEGATIVE HABITS

There is no denying we really are creatures of habit. Our habits enable us to complete simple tasks automatically without having to think too deeply. When considering current habits and looking to create new ones, it's important to think about the impact these habits have on us. Are there any habits that rule your life? How do they make you feel? Habits that have a positive impact and bring you closer to your goals are the ones to hone. Anything that has a negative impact on your life and drains your energy should be eliminated.

In 1960, Dr Maxwell Maltz proposed a theory that remains popular today. He argued that it takes 21 days to form a habit and 90 days to make it permanent. Bear this in mind when making lifestyle changes and don't give up too easily.

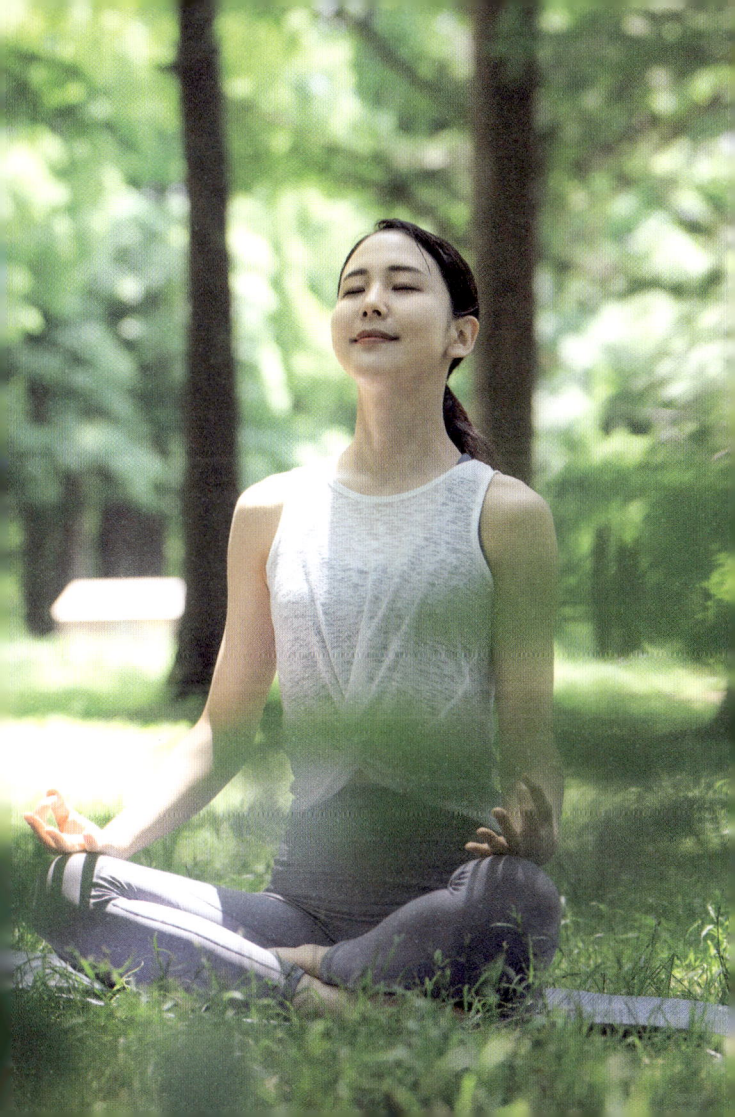

MAKING THE HABIT STICK

It's easy to implement a new habit, but ensuring it becomes a permanent part of your daily routine can be much trickier. It's important to be realistic about how much spare time you have to devote to this practice. If you're keen to try journalling, try a bit of free writing each night before you go to bed. To get started, simply start writing whatever comes to mind and don't stop. It doesn't matter how mundane or insignificant – what you ate for lunch, what you need to do tomorrow – if you keep writing, the profound stuff will come. Set a timer for however long you like – 2, 5 or 10 minutes and leave a notebook and pen by your bed as a reminder.

When practised regularly, journalling can have a positive effect on your mental outlook. You can eventually build more time into this activity to allow for lengthier sessions.

Beginning is easy.
Continuing is hard.

JAPANESE PROVERB

SETTING GOALS

Some people refer to ikigai as "their reason to get up in the morning". The start of the day is the best time to begin your practice.

Instead of reaching for your phone as soon as you wake up, turn it off or set it to silent mode. Take a moment to choose an action or activity that will bring you joy today. Perhaps it's going for a run or doing some yoga; maybe some time with a book or lunch with a friend. Take a moment to think about this intention and visualize how you can make it happen. By making the decision to do something joyful for yourself and mindfully going through the steps of how to make it happen, you are not only more likely to achieve it and boost your mood, but the act of making the decision will help you feel more in control and likely shape the course of your day.

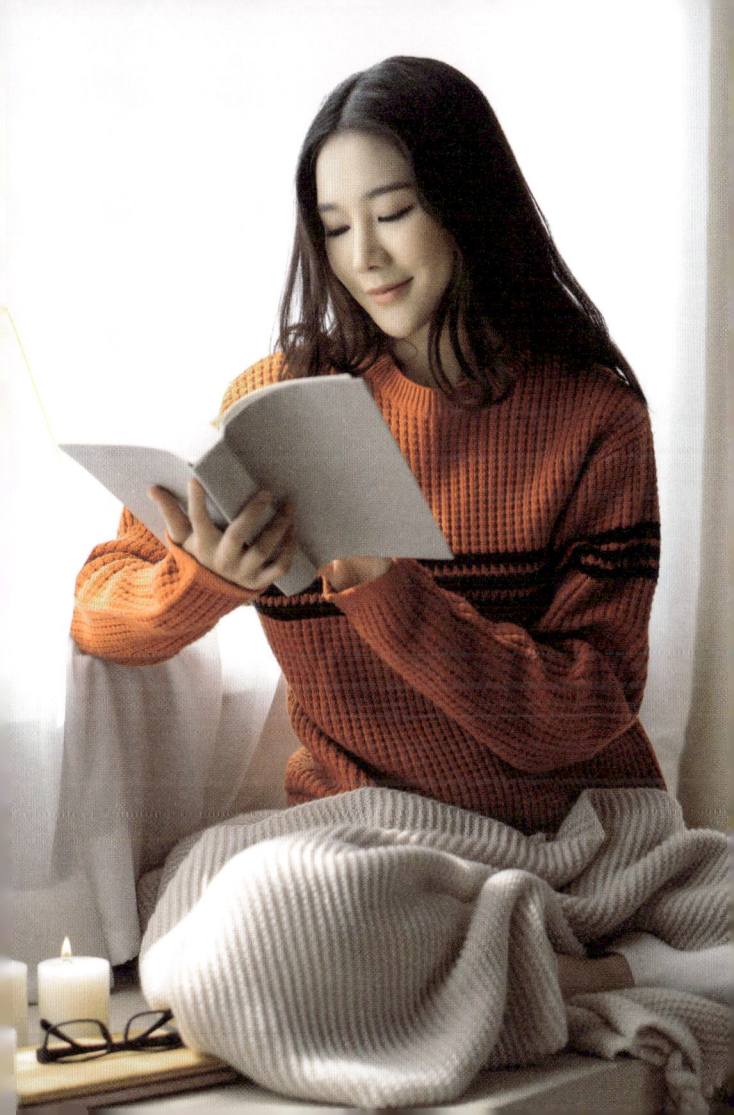

SELF-REFLECTION

Life can fly by at breakneck speed allowing little or no time for us to pause for thought. While self-reflection is something most of us do in our day-to-day lives, doing it consciously is a way to fulfil your ikigai. It can be incredibly beneficial to set aside a quiet moment to run through recent life events and changes, take stock and think about what's working and what isn't. We can end up going along with things that don't work because we don't have the time to think how we could approach the situation in a different way, leading us to feel frustrated.

By reflecting on the processes and happenings, we can analyze our lives and make changes for the better. No matter how small, each positive change is a step forward on your ikigai journey. By making a series of small, positive changes, you'll cover a lot of ground in no time.

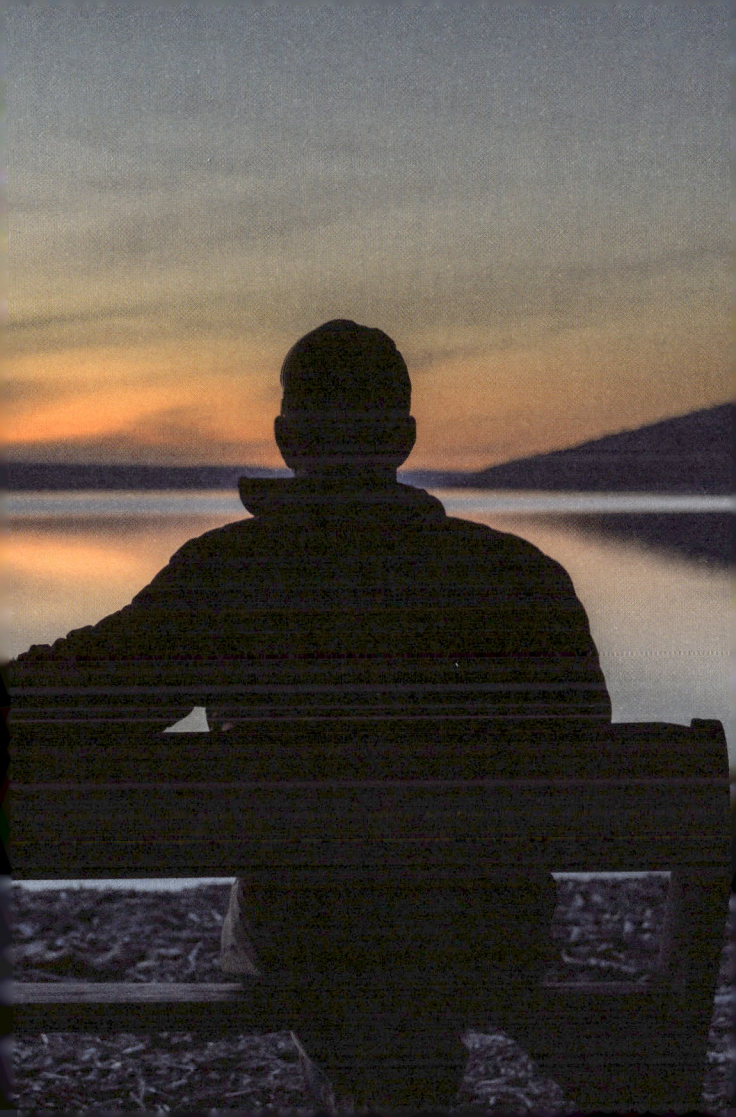

WRITING A
GRATITUDE JOURNAL

As well as looking for areas you want to change, reflecting on the things that make you happy can guide you towards your ikigai. A very simple daily practice to help you look for the positives in your life is to keep a gratitude journal.

The best time to write a gratitude journal is last thing at night. Try to do this every night and always write in the same notebook so you can look back as you make progress.

Take a couple of minutes to reflect on your day and write down three things you feel grateful for. These could be as small as a delicious new sandwich you discovered, or as big as the unfaltering support of a partner or friend; perhaps you're grateful for your work or living situation today, or that you managed to take some time for yourself.

Writing down things you feel grateful for helps retrain your brain to look to the positive rather than the negative, and to do so in your day-to-day life.

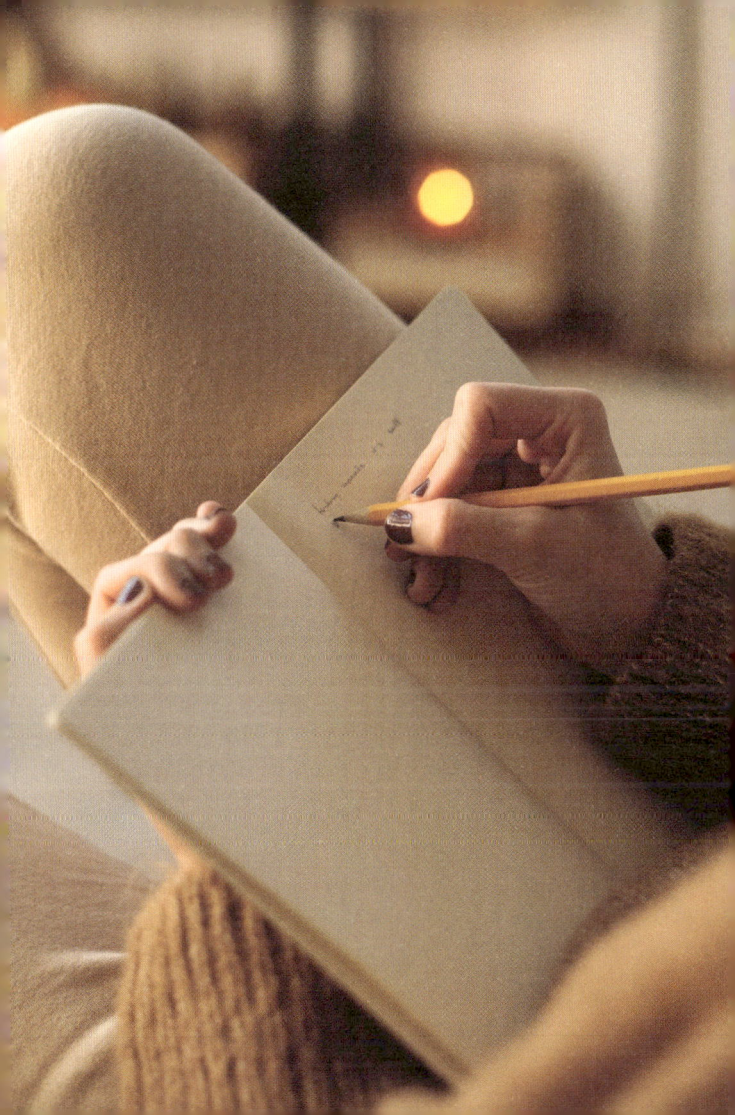

MEDITATION

Meditation is incredibly useful for focusing your mind to achieve clarity. Tried and tested techniques promote concentration and redirect unwanted or negative thoughts so you can be more aware of the present moment and achieve a sense of peace through your mind and body.

The great thing about meditation is that you can do it anywhere that you can sit comfortably and for any amount of time. Start by meditating for just a couple of minutes each day and build up to longer to achieve a state of deeper relaxation and sense of contentment.

The more you meditate, the easier you will find it to find a place of concentration and focus, where the present moment is all that matters. Use the time that follows your meditation to have clear and concise thoughts about your ikigai journey and what you can do to further yourself along the path.

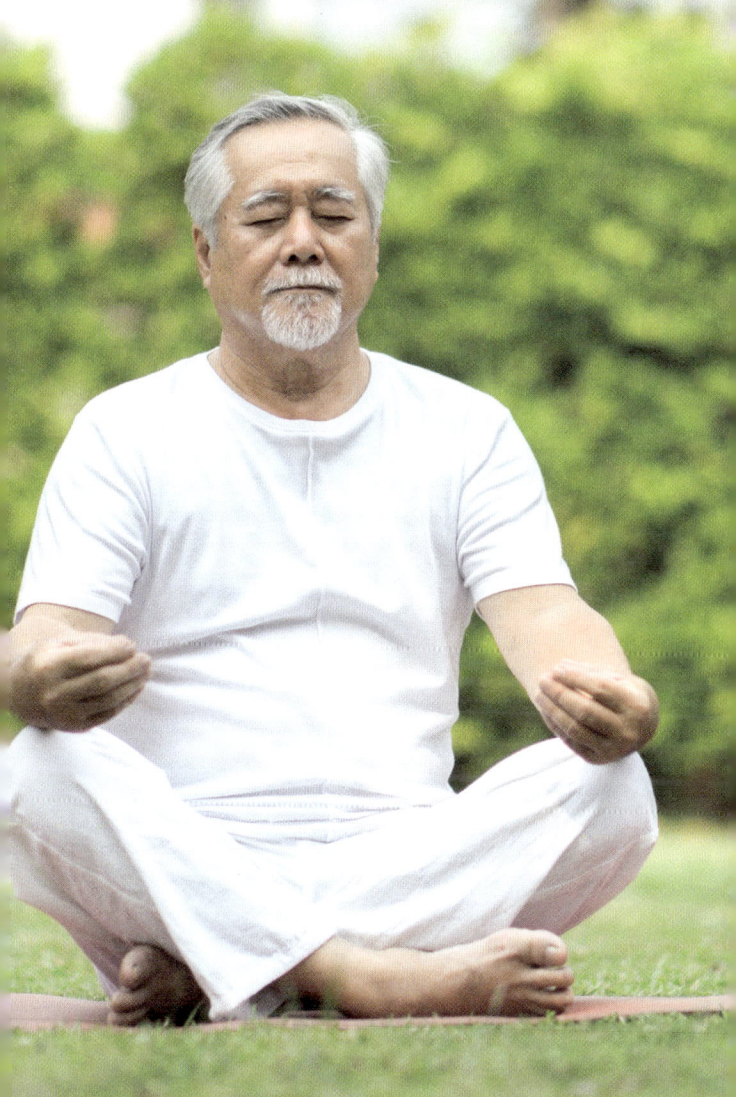

MEDITATION EXERCISE

Find somewhere quiet where you won't be disturbed. Either sit or lie down and get comfortable – the aim is to be still throughout, so make sure you're in a position you can stay in for as long as you plan to meditate. If this is your first time meditating, set a time limit – 5–10 minutes is a good place to start.

Relax and roll your shoulders to prepare. Then close your eyes and focus on your breath as you breathe in and out.

It's natural for your mind to wander, but when it does, return your focus to your breath. You might find counting the seconds you spend breathing in and out helps you refocus.

When your time is up, open your eyes, sit for a moment and notice how you feel, before getting up and continuing with your day.

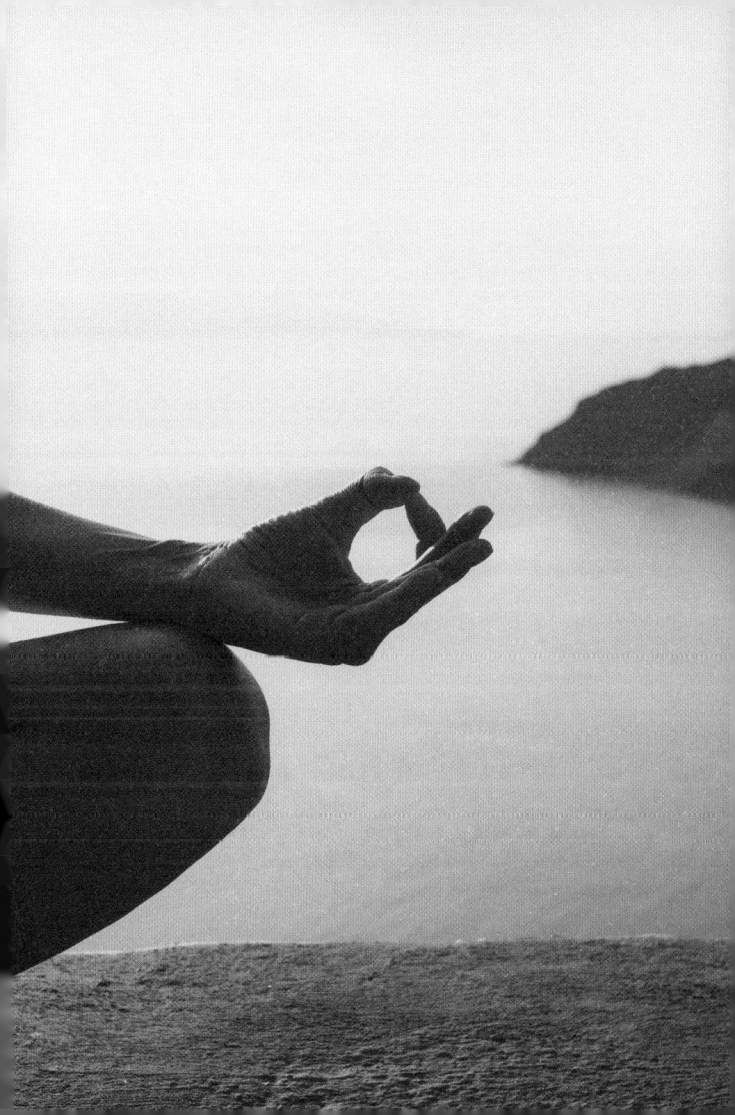

MINDFULNESS

Mindfulness is about harnessing your awareness of the present moment, without judgement, using your senses. It involves training your brain to focus on the present and pull your thoughts back to it if your mind wanders. Mindfulness can be practised anywhere at any time, which makes it easy to incorporate into your daily routine. Habit-forming is key to ikigai and these small acts of mindfulness will ultimately help you relax and take more enjoyment from life situations.

Try practising mindfulness while you're eating or drinking. Pay attention to the taste, texture and temperature of what you are eating or drinking: how does it feel on your tongue or when you swallow? When you're in the shower, close your eyes and think about how the water feels as it lands on your skin. How does the temperature feel? Stand still and listen to the continuous sound of the water as it pours out of the shower. Does it make you feel a sense of calm?

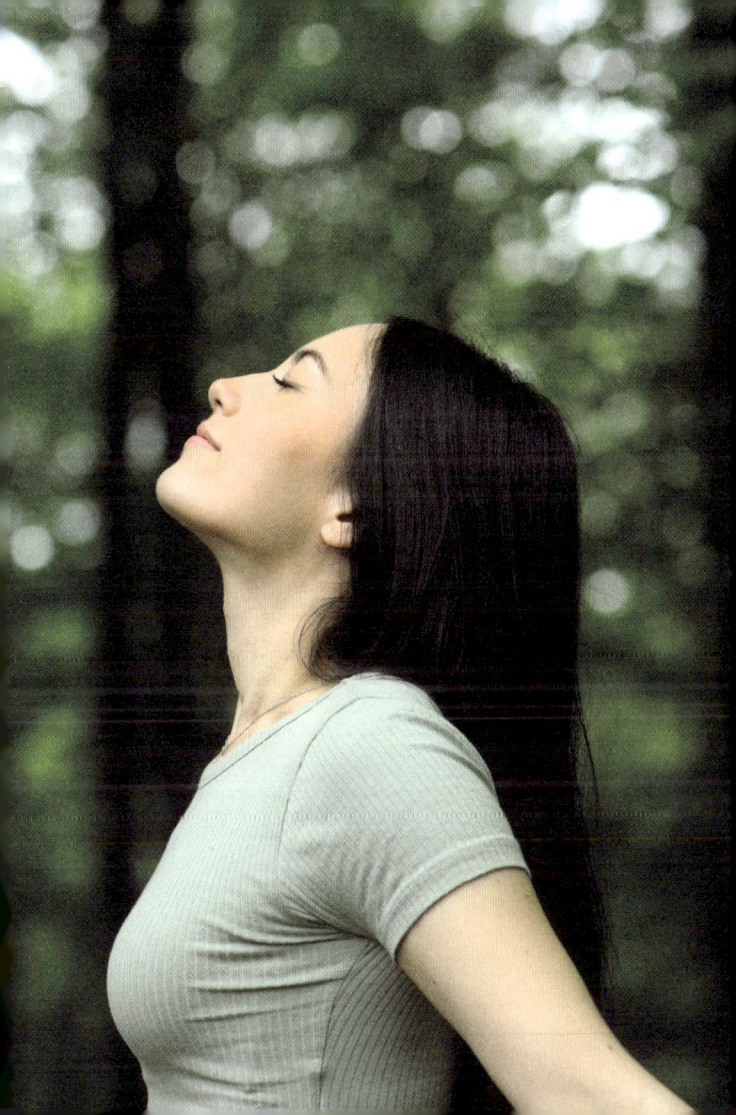

MINDFULNESS EXERCISE

A good place to start is with a body scan.

Lie down on your bed or sofa and get comfortable. Take a few deep breaths and when you start to relax you can begin.

Shift your attention to your body. Starting from the top of your head, stop to focus on each part of your body, slowly scanning all the way down to your toes, paying attention to how everything feels. What sensations do you notice? Are you holding tension in any part of your body? Do any parts feel more relaxed than others? Take in all the aches, pains, tingles and other feelings, all while lying perfectly still.

This relaxing exercise will help focus your mind for any tasks ahead, as you continue to strive for purpose and make progress in your search for ikigai.

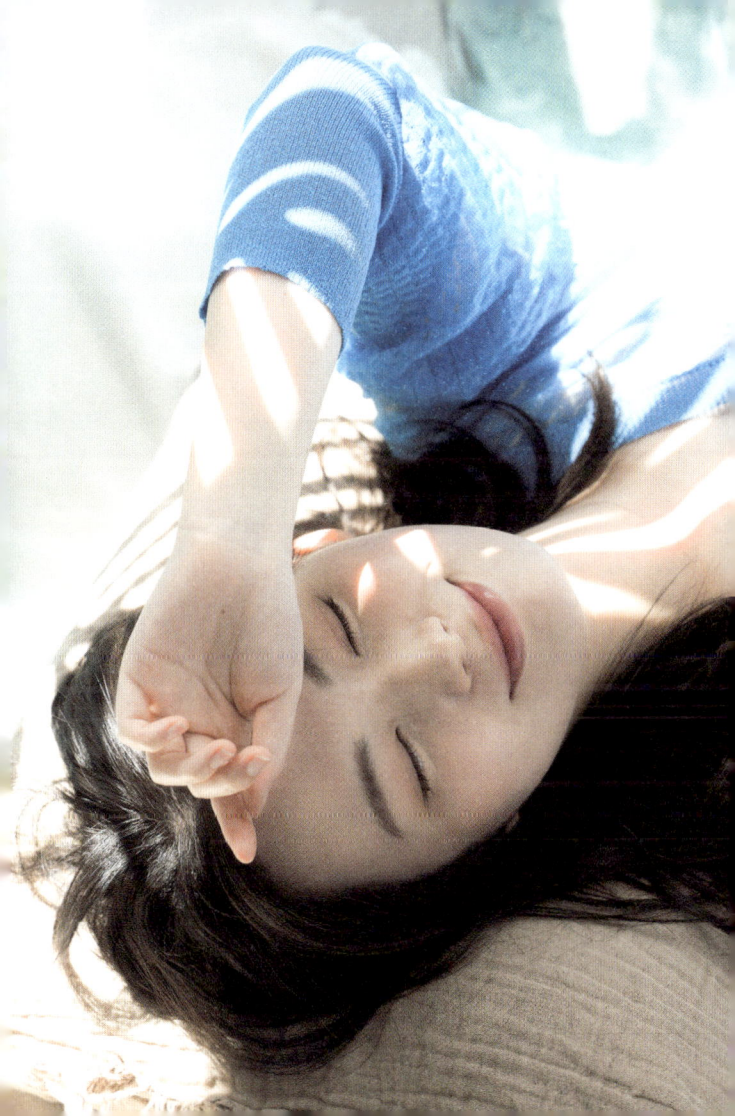

VISUALIZATION

While visualization has historically had mystical connotations, in more modern times it is viewed as a meditative self-help tool, used to help you reach your goals. As we saw on page 62, setting goals is incredibly helpful on your journey to finding your ikigai.

Visualization is all about creating an image in your mind of where you would like to be in life and engaging your senses to really "feel" it. The idea is that by encouraging yourself into a certain mindset, you can work towards and eventually reach the goal you have visualized.

There are two different types of visualization: outcome visualization involves thinking about what you would like to happen and envisioning the end result, while process visualization is about envisioning each step towards your outcome. These two practices can be used together for even stronger results. Try the exercise on page 78.

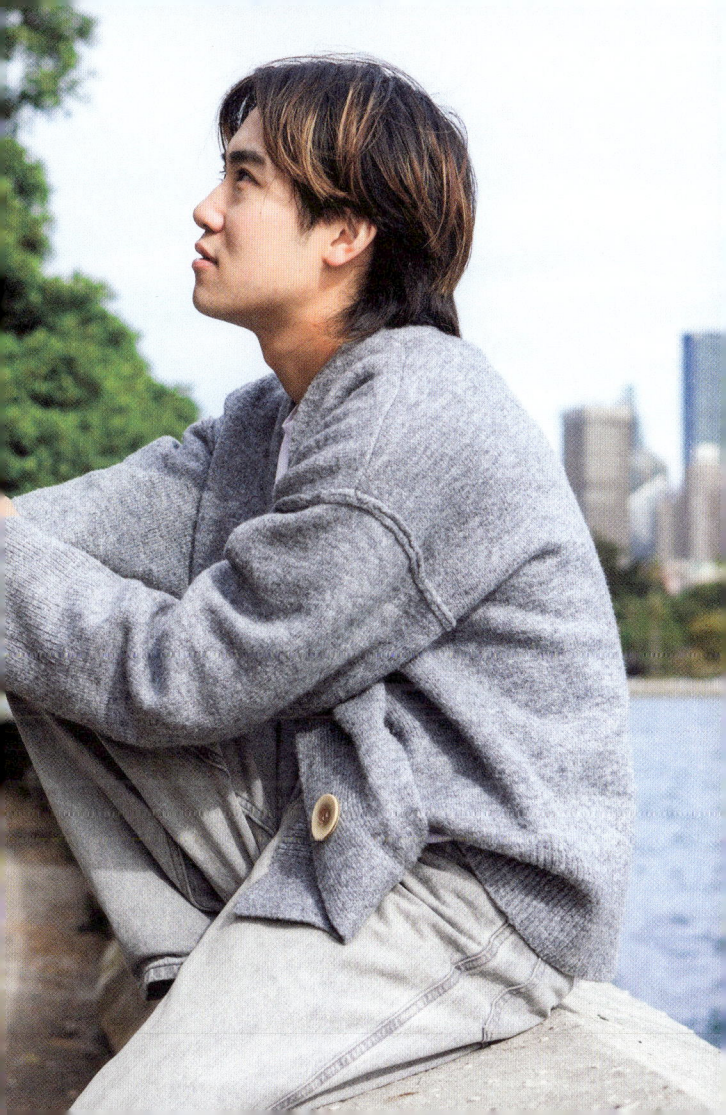

VISUALIZATION EXERCISE

As well as helping you work towards your goals, visualization aids relaxation and calms the mind. Try this exercise to get into a headspace that will help you make life decisions and strive for that all-important ikigai.

Find a comfortable place to sit. Close your eyes. Take some time to get into the right frame of mind. Focus on your breathing, taking long breaths in and out to calm your nervous system. Then, visualize something you would like to achieve or change in your life – perhaps you would like to move to a new home, for example. Take your mind through the steps to achieving this. Visualize yourself being handed the keys. Imagine what your new home smells and feels like. How do you feel?

Practise this regularly to see life from a different perspective and unleash new ideas.

Passion is energy.
Feel the power that
comes from focusing on
what excites you.

OPRAH WINFREY

AFFIRMATIONS

Affirmations are positive phrases that, when practised regularly, can help shift negative thought patterns you might have in a more favourable direction. Not only will these nuggets of positivity help instantly boost your mood when you need a pick-me-up, but this form of positive thinking can help rewire your brain, giving you a fresh perspective in certain situations and supporting you with ikigai-related life changes.

Affirmations are phrases that you choose or devise and should be selected to suit your situation. Repeating them to yourself in the mirror first thing in the morning is a good place to start. Perhaps you've started a new job and you're feeling a little out of your depth. You might say to yourself, "I am confident and capable." If you're trying to live a more fulfilled life, you might choose, "I deserve happiness and success."

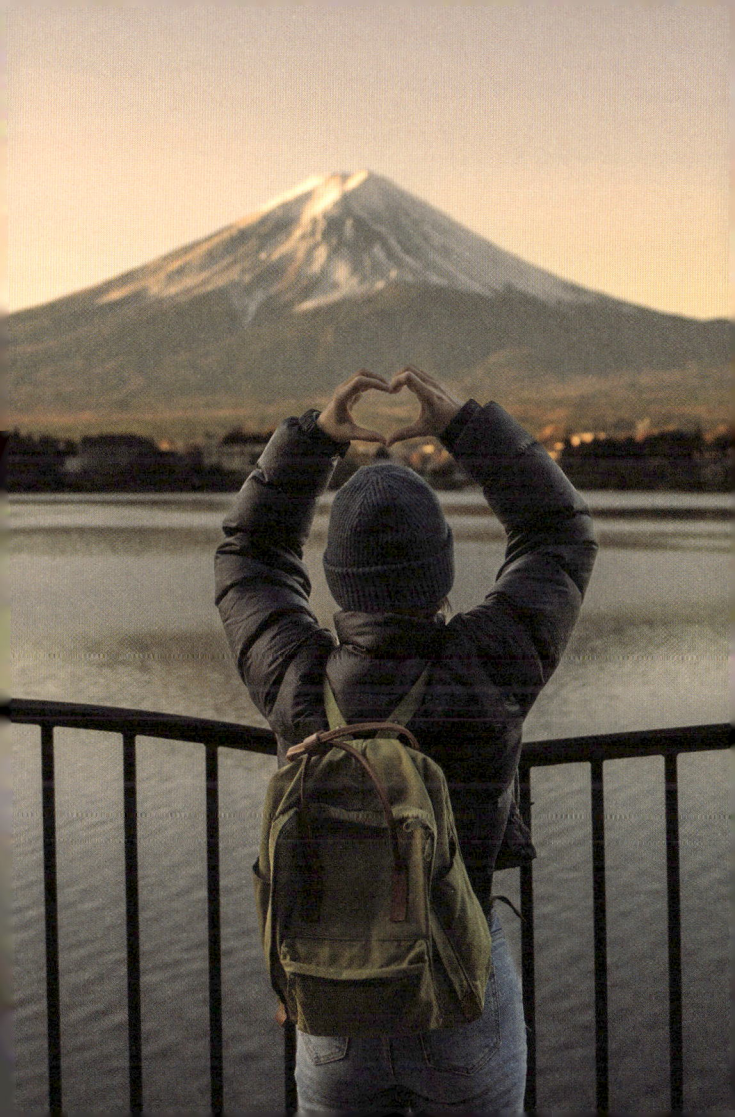

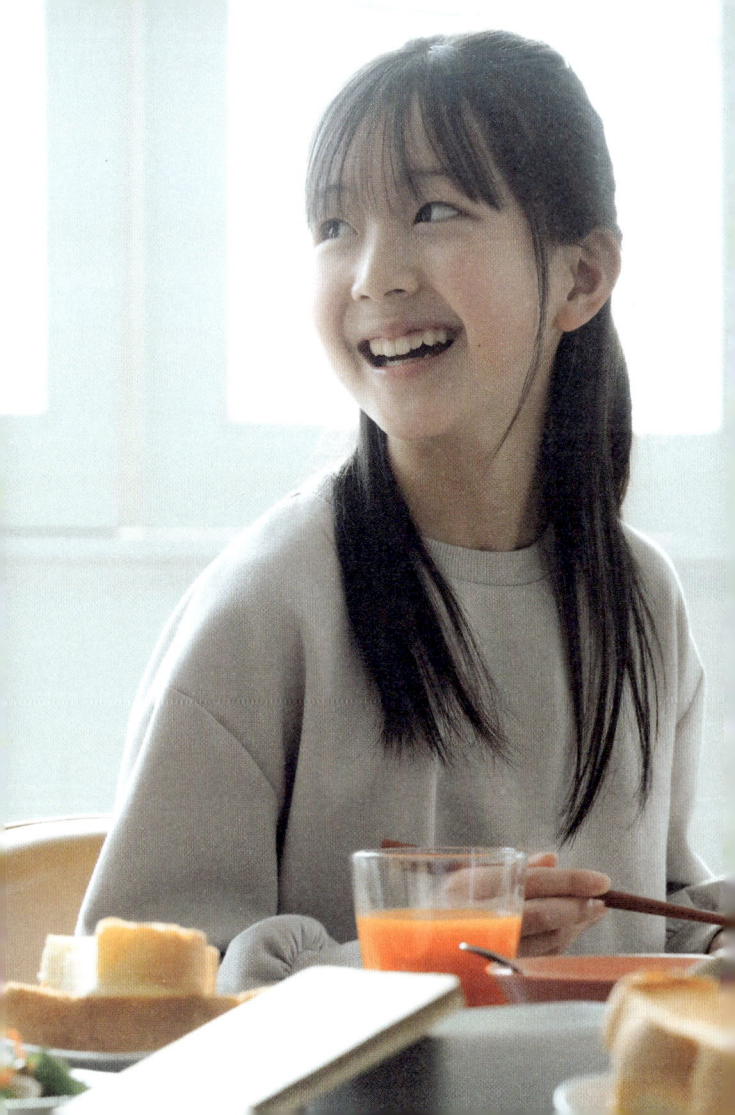

THE 80 PER CENT RULE

One of the practices associated with ikigai is eating until you are 80 per cent full. This stems from a common saying in Japanese, often said before or after a meal: "Hara hachi bu." This translates as "fill your belly to 80 per cent." In *Ikigai: The Japanese Secret to a Long and Happy Life*, García and Miralles found this to be widely practised by Okinawans. It is believed this spares their digestive system the lengthy processing of food that causes cellular oxidation, which can damage cells over time.

Learning when your body is 80 per cent full can be tricky. The advice is to try to stop eating when you start to feel full. The idea is that eschewing the extras we might usually have with our meals – and the bonus snacks throughout the day – brings about long-term health benefits and helps us learn self-discipline.

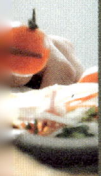

FOREST BATHING

The importance of the natural world to our mental and physical well-being can't be overestimated. Heading outside for some fresh air can provide clarity of mind when searching for our ikigai, as well as bringing incomparable health benefits.

The Japanese have a term for the practice of immersing oneself in nature to bring about healing. *Shinrin-yoku* – widely referred to in the West as "forest bathing" – is a term originally introduced by the Japanese Ministry for Agriculture in the 1980s in an effort to encourage people to spend time outdoors.

Just being out in the fresh air – in sun, rain or the breeze – can have therapeutic benefits, and if you are surrounded by plants and greenery, the rewards are even greater.

While forest bathing is all about deepening your connection with nature by immersing yourself in the outside world, you can also reap the benefits by having natural wood and green, leafy plants in your home.

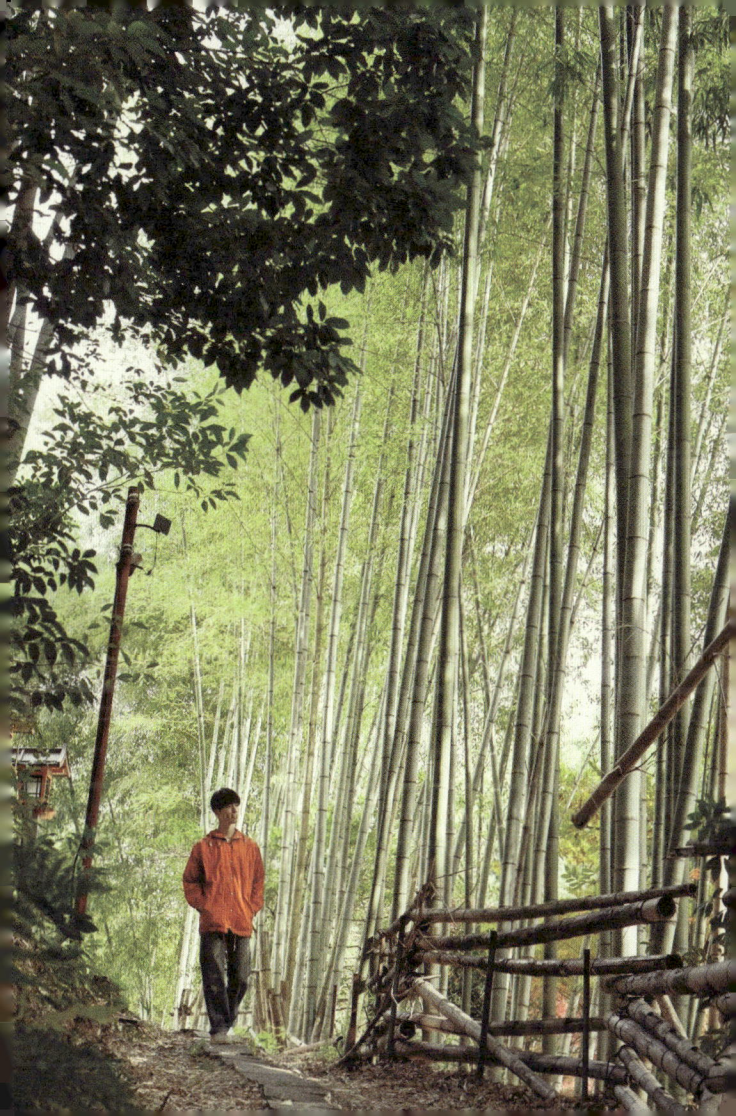

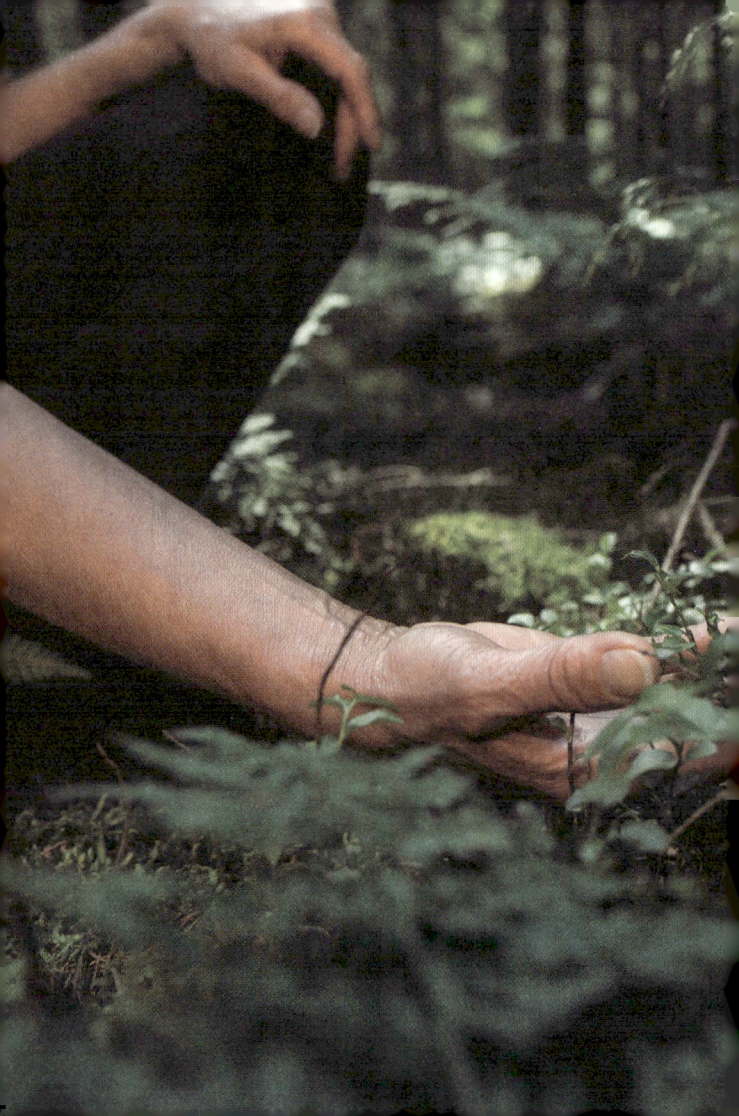

FOREST BATHING EXERCISE

Take some time out of your day to visit a green space near where you live. This can be a park, garden, woodland or forest – as long as there is enough greenery to help you feel connected to nature, you will feel the benefits of this practice.

Spend time alone and experience your surroundings through your various senses. Mindfully study the plants – their leaves, branches and flowers – do you notice anything that you might not have before? Run your fingers over the plants and consider their texture – soft moss and rough branches will provide different sensations – what does the softness of a flower's petals remind you of?

Close your eyes and listen – how many different sounds can you hear? Which can you recognize? With your eyes still closed, take a deep breath through your nose and fill your lungs with the scent of your surroundings. Which smells do you recognize? How do these individual sensations make you feel?

YOGA

Yoga offers far-reaching benefits for both mind and body, from improving muscle strength, tone and posture, to boosting energy, promoting circulation and restorative sleep, and creating an overall sense of calm and relaxation. You are likely to find yoga useful as you search for your ikigai; not only will it offer clarity of mind, but also it will help you feel good, encouraging you to seek enjoyment in more areas of your life.

There are many different styles of yoga – from the faster-paced hot and flow styles; to mindful Hatha and Ashtanga, which balance head, heart and body; and the more passive yin, to release tension and heal the nervous system. With so much choice you will find something to suit you, enabling you to move at your own pace.

You can practise yoga in the comfort of your home, using books and online videos for reference.

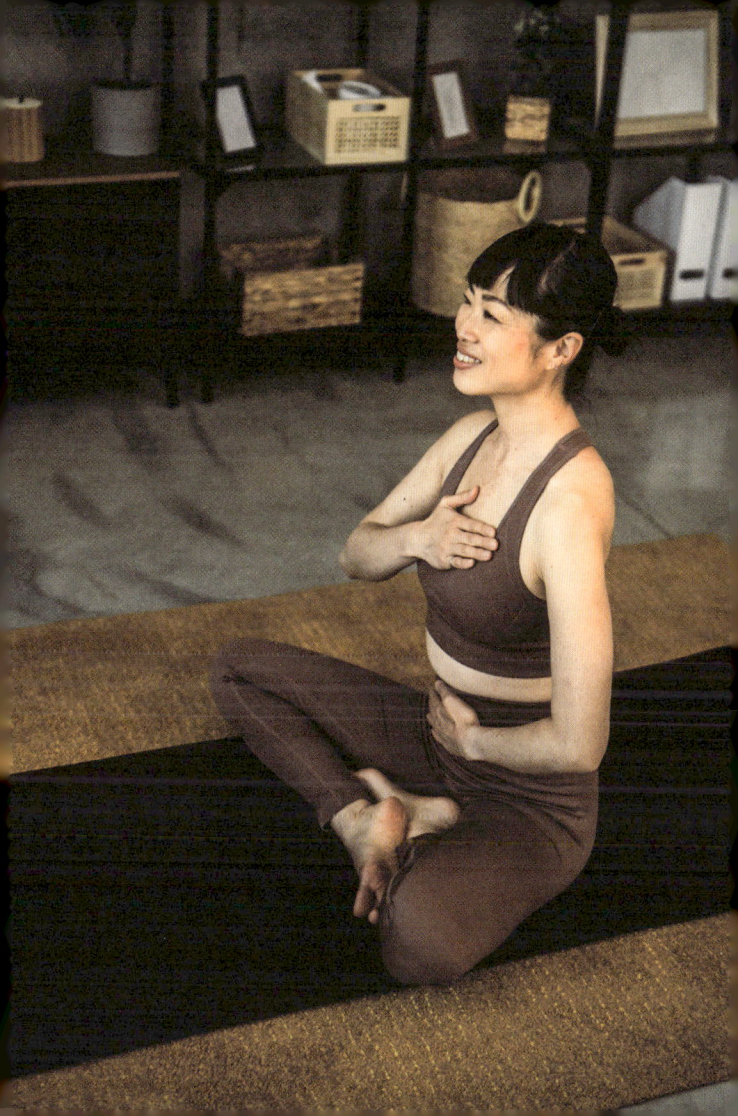

WALKING

It sounds so simple but walking somewhere when you might otherwise have jumped in the car or onto a bus can have a hugely positive effect on your mental and physical health. Research shows that fresh air increases oxygen levels to your brain, which in turn raises serotonin levels, helping your body to relax and feel calm. Natural light helps regulate our sleep/wake cycles and vitamin D from the sunlight will help give a further serotonin boost.

Boosting happiness levels and getting the most enjoyment out of life that you can is what the ikigai journey is all about.

Even better than simply walking to work or the shops, for a further boost take yourself for a longer walk in pleasant, green surroundings. Your brain and your body will thank you for it!

*Only staying active
will make you want to
live a hundred years.*

JAPANESE PROVERB

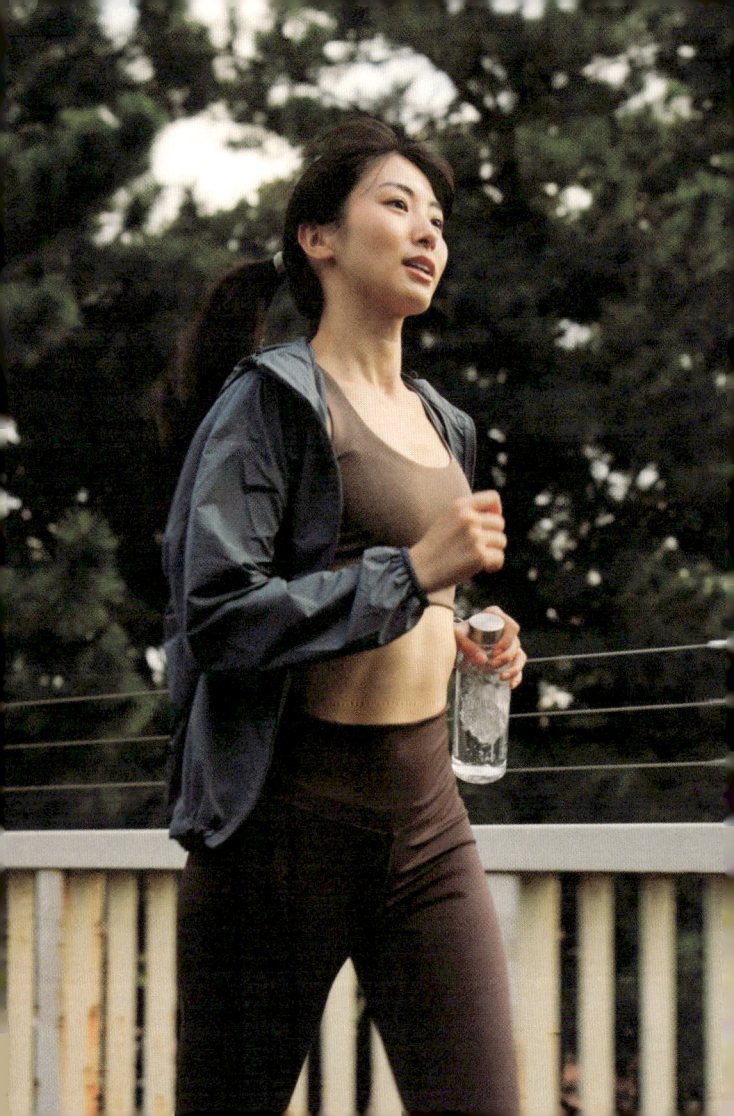

RUNNING

Whether you run for an hour or 10 minutes, there are few easier, cheaper or better ways to give your brain an instant boost. As long as you have a pair of running shoes and are physically able to do so, you can step out of your front door and run to the end of the road and back a few times at no financial cost to you and very little cost to your precious time. As well as the obvious health benefits, running will help fuel a go-getting attitude when it comes to harnessing your ikigai.

Consider signing up to an organized run – it doesn't have to be a long one. Collecting sponsorship money for a charity close to your heart can be a good motivation, as well as contributing to your ikigai journey by offering something the world needs. Setting a goal with a deadline can really help in reaching it.

NEW HOBBIES

Making time in your schedule to try new hobbies can really help you connect with your ikigai. There are so many hobbies and activities out there you've never tried before that could bring you great enjoyment, propelling you ever further on your ikigai journey as you seek joy and purpose in life.

Start with an activity you've thought about doing but never managed to fit in and see where that takes you. Join a class, learn from online tutorials or ask a friend to teach you something. You could be even bolder and pick something you haven't considered before – it could just be your true calling!

No matter what stage you are at in your life, it's never too late to learn something new. And once you've mastered it, perhaps you could teach others and continue your ikigai journey in that way.

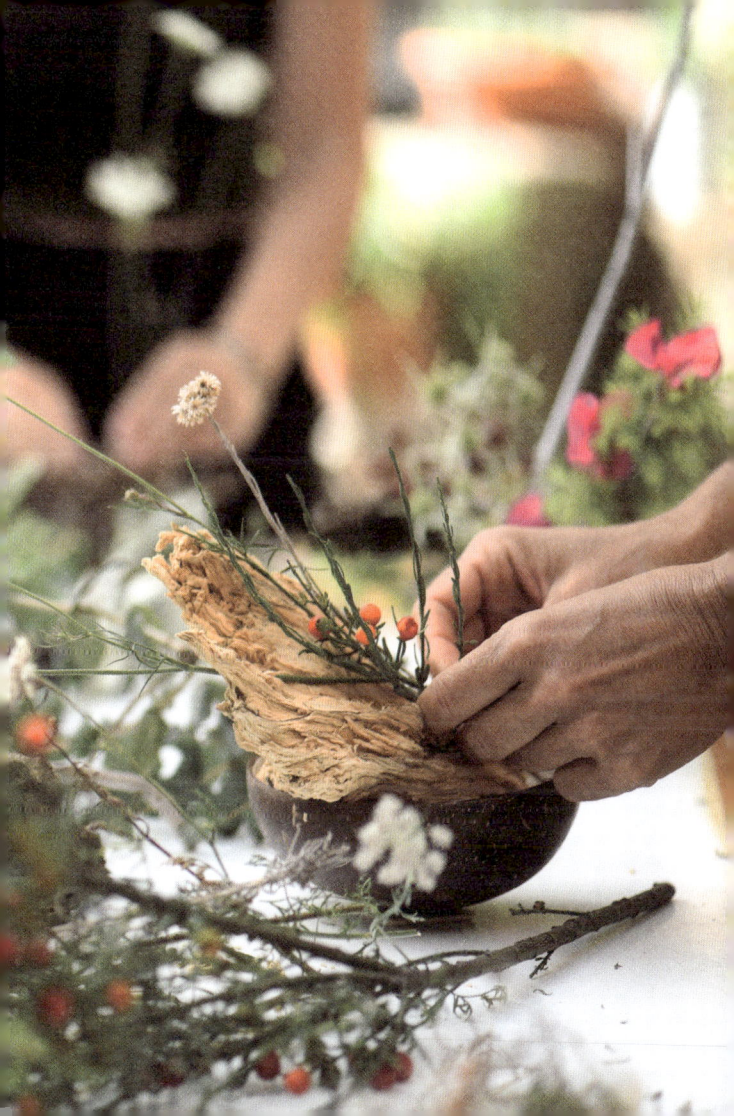

NEXT STEPS TO IKIGAI

Following the advice in this chapter will likely have left you with more room to think and an understanding of how having time for yourself will help you find your ikigai. Whether you find yourself drawn to meditation, running or focused hobbies, spend 5 minutes after each session writing down any thoughts you might have had while doing these activities. The headspace you find through exercise and mindful wellness practices is incredibly valuable and helps bring about creative thinking.

Ikigai involves both a long-term process and a series of small changes to your daily life, so it's also important to keep an open mind – as the next chapter explains, your ikigai will evolve with you and keeping pace with it is key to harnessing its full potential.

TO FIND YOUR
IKIGAI IS TO
FIND YOUR
JOY IN LIFE

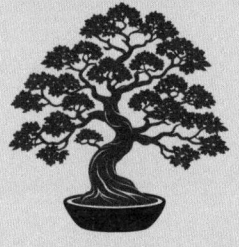

LIVING
WITH
IKIGAI

So, you've found your ikigai or you are on the right path to discovering it. This is fantastic news! This chapter suggests ways to maintain your ikigai and keep the momentum going through the areas of your life incorporated into the four pillars – what you love, what the world needs, what you are good at and what you can be paid for.

While these areas are key, it's also important to focus on your diet, exercise and social life – these are all vital to ikigai and the search for meaning, purpose and enjoyment in your day-to-day existence. Keeping your mental and physical health in check will help the pieces of the ikigai puzzle fall into place.

So, get comfortable with prioritizing what fulfils you, keep on striving for your goals and learn to live with your newfound ikigai.

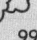

HOW TO KEEP UP
WITH IKIGAI

While finding your ikigai will feel like something to celebrate, remember it is always evolving. It could change in a few years or potentially sooner should you experience a big life event. It's also important to remember to hone your ikigai and nurture it – whatever it may be that brings you enjoyment; work hard at those relationships, strive to improve your skills or reach for that promotion if these are the things that bring you happiness.

Your ikigai journey is ongoing, with no final destination but many stops along the way; ikigai requires commitment and will span your lifetime. In Japanese culture, the word *ganbarimasu* describes the art of patience and perseverance to achieve your desired outcome. The word itself translates as "go to great lengths to achieve a goal" and is useful to have in your ikigai toolkit.

*Youthfulness of mind
is important in ikigai,
but so is commitment and
passion, however seemingly
insignificant your goal.*

KEN MOGI

ADDRESS YOUR DIET

Diet is key to a healthy lifestyle and vital to the concept of ikigai, ensuring balance and harmony in body and mind. A good place to look for advice is the centenarians of Okinawa, the birthplace of ikigai. Older islanders eat a largely plant-based diet – consisting of rice, pickles, vegetables, fish and tofu – consuming eggs and meat only occasionally, and choosing to cook and bake with olive or rapeseed oil rather than butter. The produce they eat is grown locally, ideally in their very own vegetable patch, and they traditionally give thanks before and after each meal.

As mentioned on page 82, Okinawans are mindful of how much they eat, following the 80 per cent tradition – learning to realize when your stomach is 80 per cent full and eating no more after that. This helps teach self-discipline and they reap numerous long-term health benefits.

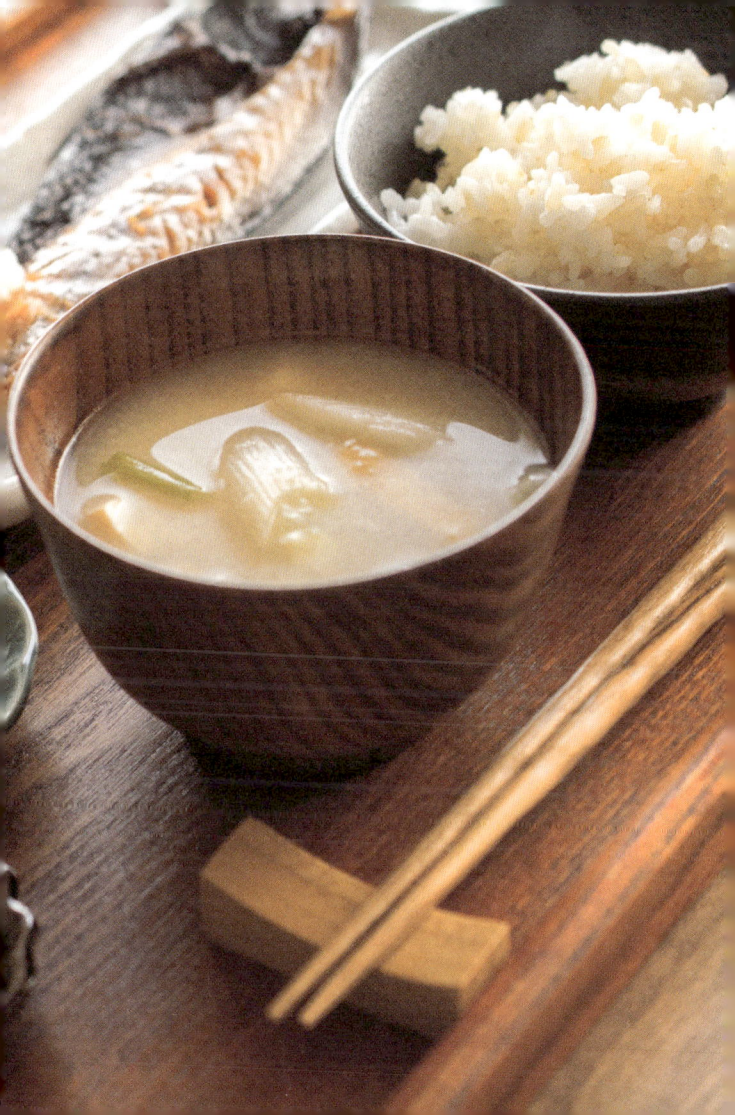

KEEP MOVING

Regular exercise is part of the essential practice of habit-forming, something that is key to maintaining your ikigai. Whether you're an adrenaline junkie or a homebody, exercise should play an important role in your life.

It's likely there is something out there to suit your mood and personality, and you can always change it up. Running and swimming can be quite mindful, giving you room to think while doing wonders for your mental and physical health. Cycling and walking can be solitary or sociable depending on how you feel; they are also likely to take you to green spaces and immerse you in nature. Team sports help you find a sense of community with like-minded people, and martial arts help you become both disciplined and focused.

Remember that exercise can be incorporated into your life in more practical ways. Could you walk to work instead of getting the bus or driving? Take the stairs instead of using the lift?

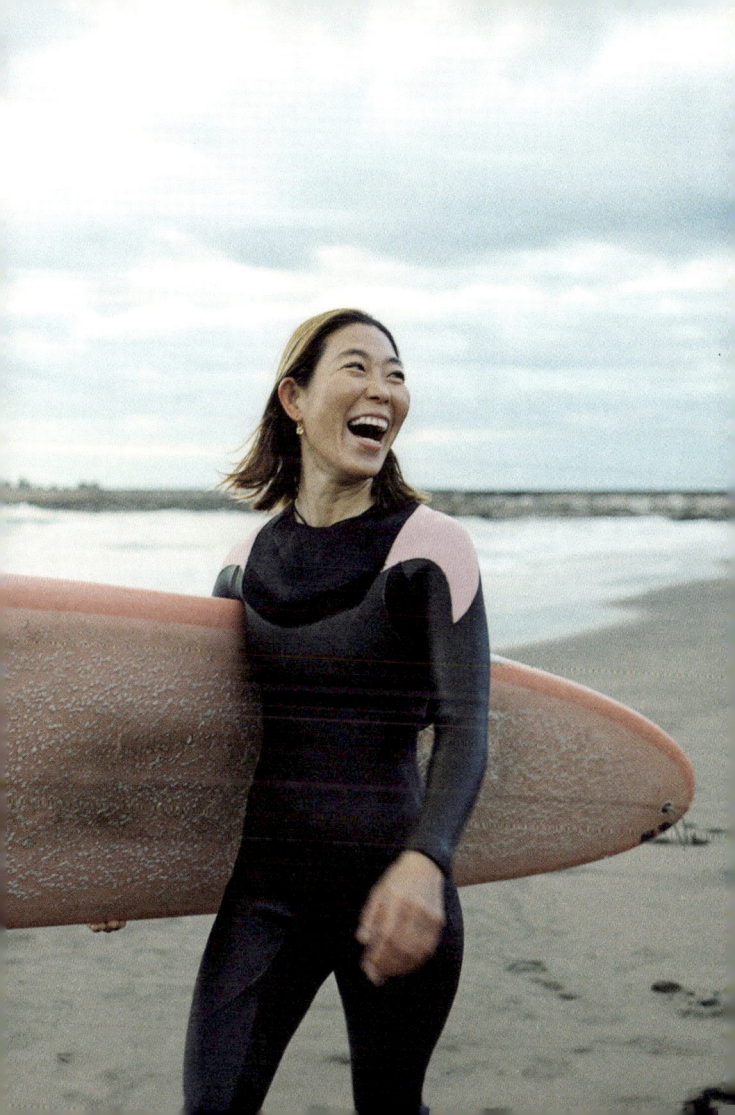

MAINTAIN
SOCIAL CONNECTIONS

Keeping in touch with friends and family is important in order to maintain good relationships and harness the enjoyment in life that you're seeking through ikigai. It will also be beneficial to your emotional health and well-being. Try not to spread yourself too thin and prioritize the friends and family who offer you support when you need it most. Make new friends, but not at the expense of the old ones who have been there for you throughout your life.

Ensure you have a healthy work–life balance but also make time to see colleagues outside of work. This element of Japanese working culture is called *nomikai* – after-work socializing that often includes drinks and karaoke. Spending time with co-workers helps you get to know them better and see who they are away from the confines of their job.

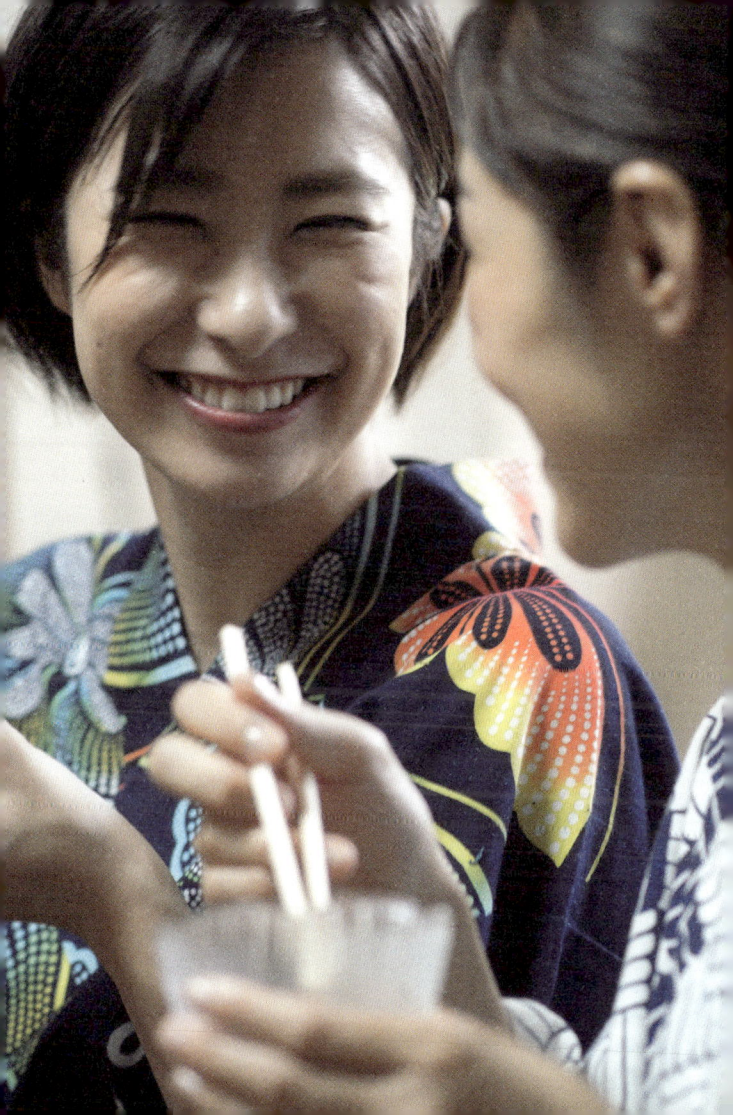

REMEMBER YOUR PASSIONS

Always remind yourself why you love the things you do. This is a great exercise to boost your mood and practise gratitude on your ikigai journey.

Take a moment to list the reasons, either in your mind or on paper. Why you love where you live, for example, or why you are grateful for your family or friendships, and how the activities, hobbies or causes you are passionate about make you feel.

It's vital you make time for the things you love, so check in with yourself regularly to ensure there's room for it all. If there isn't, reassess. The things you enjoy should not be rushed, nor should they feel like a chore. Make priority lists and ask yourself which things have a positive impact on your life and which do not.

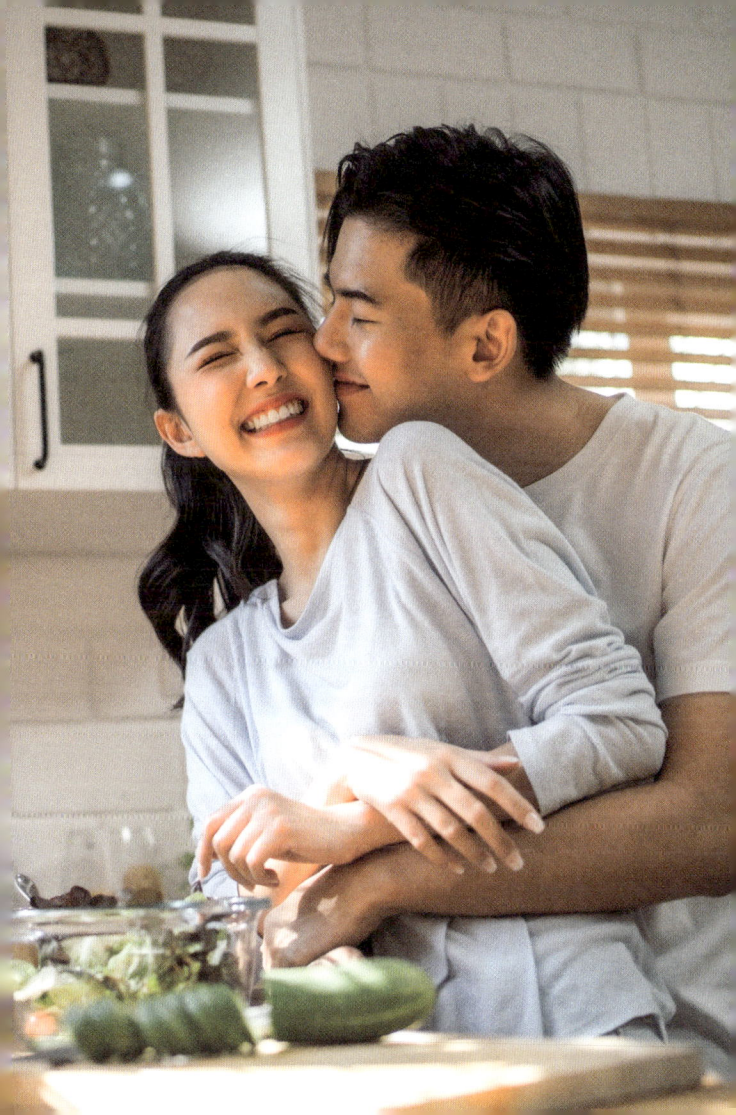

EXPLORE YOUR CREATIVE SIDE

What activities bring you joy and engage you to the point of finding your state of "flow", losing yourself in the moment? Perhaps you have a creative side and would benefit from painting, pottery, woodcraft or knitting. Perhaps these activities haven't interested you in the past, but if you are someone who likes to work with their hands and enjoys quiet moments, they are worth exploring. Don't be afraid to try new things you might have dismissed previously – as we saw in the previous chapter, new hobbies can help your ikigai to develop and hone your purpose.

Think about what you enjoy – it doesn't matter if you are skilled at it because the main purpose of ikigai is to find enjoyment in what you do. If you excel in something and it brings you joy to pursue it, even better. Whatever it is, when you make progress, you will feel a swelling sense of achievement and personal fulfilment.

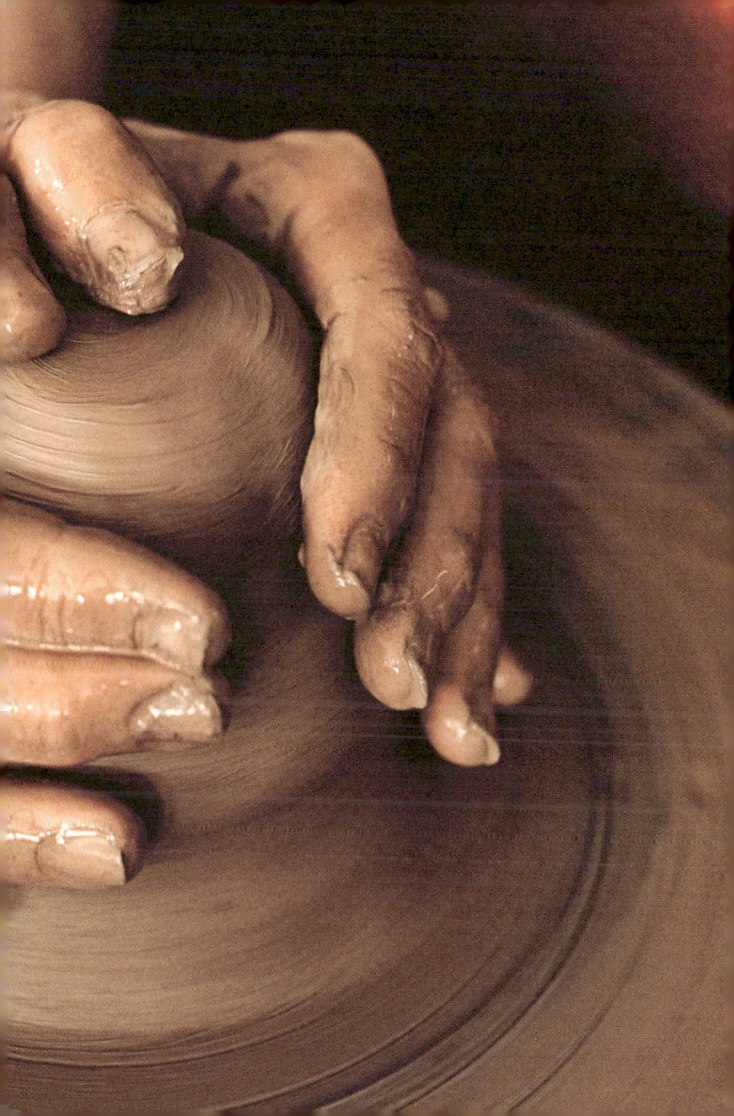

PRIORITIZE SELF-CARE

Self-care will help you achieve a positive state of mind and body – learning to love yourself is key to maintaining your ikigai. Ensuring you get enough exercise and eat well will go a long way to add to your motivation and help you achieve balance in life. By looking after yourself you will find your work is more effective and you have more energy to do the things you love.

Think about building time into your daily or weekly routine devoted to self-care or resting. This might involve some self-pampering, watching a movie or cooking. It might mean curling up with a book or meditating. It's also important to keep your brain active, so take time out to do that crossword or sudoku puzzle and, instead of reading the news online, buy a paper newspaper and find a moment to sit and read.

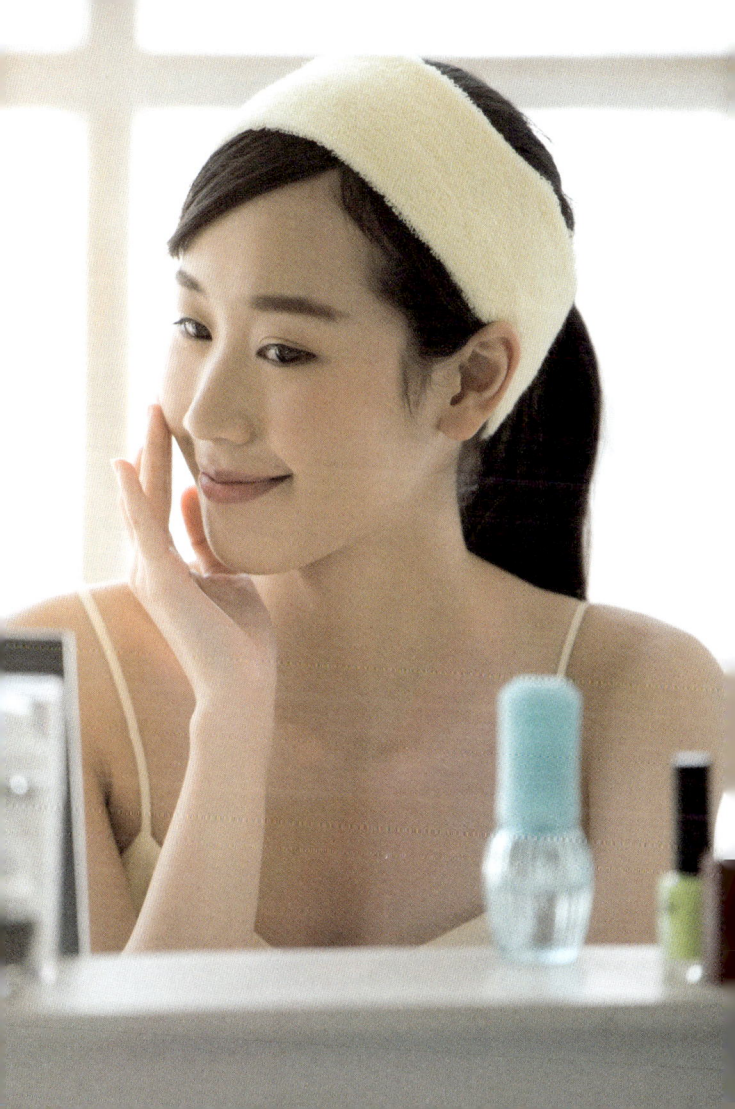

OVERCOME CHALLENGES

The path to ikigai won't always be easy and it's likely you'll face challenges along the way. Injury or ill health can hamper your ability to be active in a way you feel you need to be, and life situations might cause priorities to shift, leaving you with less time to dedicate to your ikigai journey.

It's important to stay positive and remember it won't always be like this. You will heal and your situation will evolve. Don't be afraid to ask for the help you need, sooner rather than later.

Fitting in micro-moments of self-care works wonders in lifting your mood and maintaining a sense of purpose when you feel you need it most. Try a 5- or 10-minute meditation or yoga practice or take a walk round the block to clear your head. Your ikigai journey doesn't have to halt because life gets in the way.

*People cannot change
their habits without
first changing their
way of thinking.*

MARIE KONDO

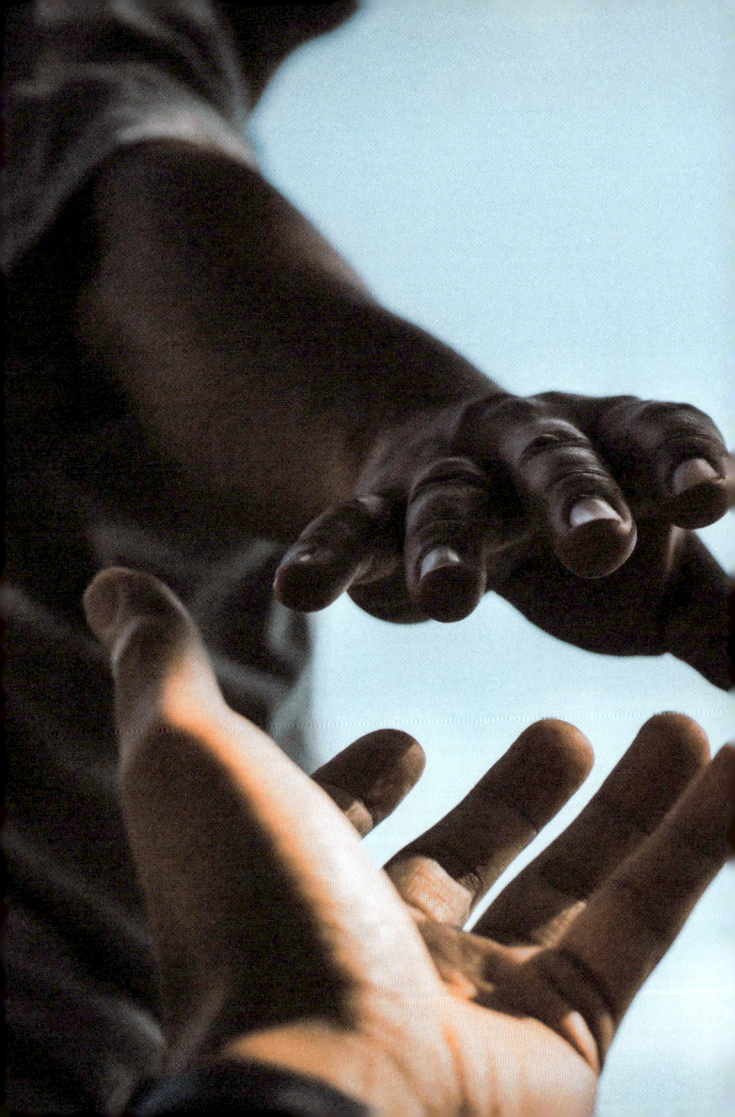

MAINTAIN YOUR CONTRIBUTION

Thinking about what the world needs – whether that means consuming mindfully, volunteering or standing up for what you believe in – should always be on your mind. Your contribution to the world is essential to your ikigai and is something you need to keep up to maintain your sense of purpose.

Start local and look for opportunities to help others within your community; don't feel you have to save the world single-handed. You will find yourself drawn to like-minded others and find further strength in numbers. Start small and bigger things will follow. If opportunities dry up in one area, look to others for ways you can help and make a difference. Joining groups of others who share your world views and desire to help – whether on social media or face to face within your community – will inspire you to keep up with the issues close to your heart.

FIND YOUR CAUSE

If you're not sure how or where to look in terms of offering help, here are some ideas. There are many different ways you can make a difference.

- Look up local charities – they will always need volunteers, whether for events, retail or fundraising.
- Take part in a sponsored sporting event, choosing a charity close to your heart to support.
- Volunteer at a food bank or help collect items for refugees. This is a very worthy use of your time.
- Offer to listen to those who need help and advice, whether via a helpline or through a mentoring scheme.
- Donate your time to keep the elderly company or read to those who can no longer manage it themselves – or to children at the local library or school.
- Take part in a beach clean or litter pick in the local park.
- Volunteer at a homeless shelter or take part in a demonstration in support of something you feel strongly about.

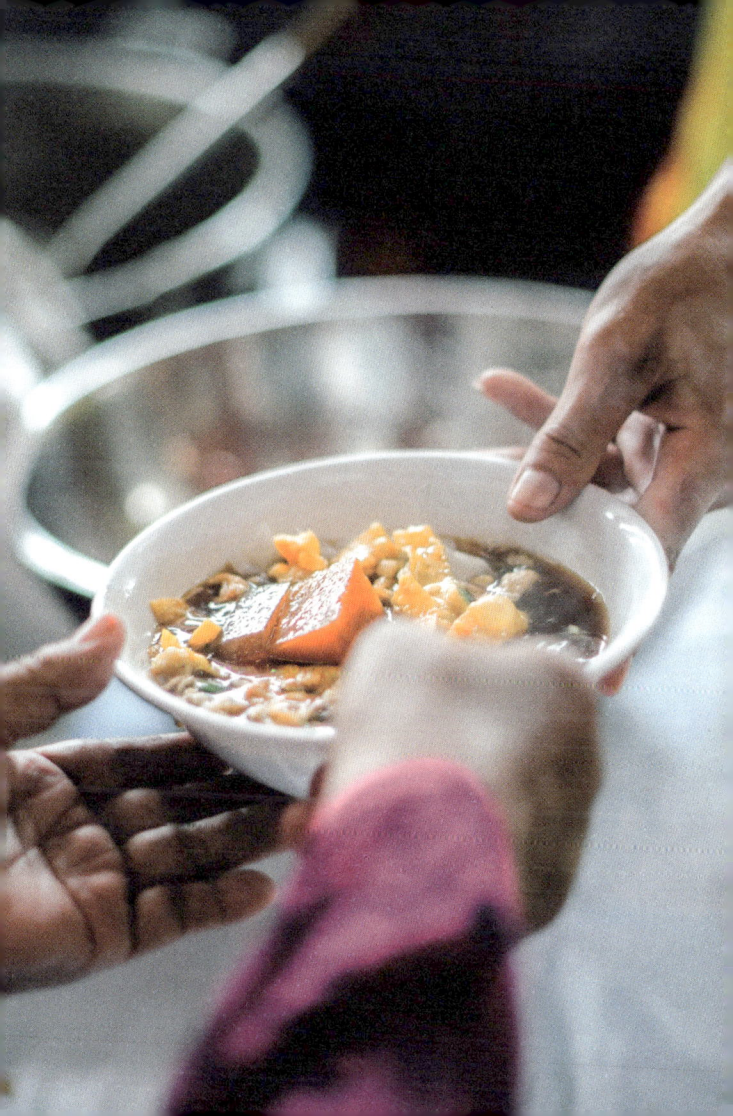

CONNECT WITH
YOUR CORE VALUES

Assessing your core values and outlining what is most important to you is a good way to align your beliefs with a cause that feels worthy. Perhaps you are an animal lover and would like to work with an animal charity – either caring for the creatures or by fundraising – or you'd like to be a human representative for our friends in the animal kingdom and fight for rights on their behalf.

Maybe you wear your politics on your sleeve and have always wanted to join a demonstration or lead an online petition. Perhaps changes in infrastructure within your local community, such as a new road through a nature reserve, don't represent progress for you, and you want to protest. Or thinking lovingly about lost grandparents makes you want to read to the elderly. Grab the bull by the horns and get involved now rather than regretting it later. Contributing to the world – via your local community or otherwise – is integral to your ikigai journey.

*The purpose of life
is a life of purpose.*

ROBERT BYRNE

KEEP PURSUING
YOUR TALENTS

The Japanese concept for the art of continuous improvement is *kaizen*, which translates as "change for the better". This philosophy encourages you to continue evolving your skills and talents through small but meaningful changes. This helps you as your ikigai evolves and takes on new meaning throughout your life.

Think about where you can improve and expand, and little by little, you will find yourself getting more effective at what you do. This can apply to a hobby, talent or your job. The idea is to always try and think creatively, be on the lookout for solutions and be proactive in your approach.

When it comes to your skills, try to focus on a couple of core strengths rather than spreading yourself too thinly across too many things. This will give you the space and discipline you need to maintain your evolving ikigai.

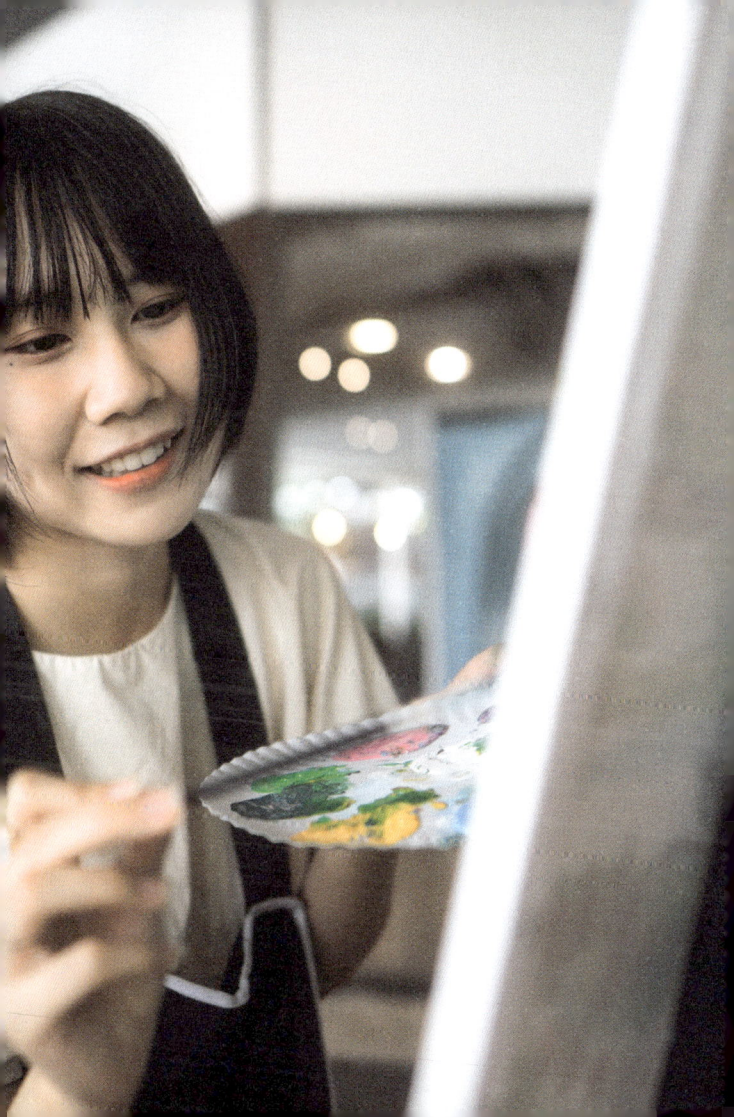

FIND ENJOYMENT
THROUGH YOUR TALENTS

Although some people are more privileged than others in being able to explore their talents, we can create our own opportunities to explore ours. Some skills come and go as we age or as our lives change course, so it's important to remember that you are seeking enjoyment here – the key to maintaining your ikigai. Be careful about pushing yourself into something that doesn't benefit you in this way.

Make a list of things you enjoy and think about how to incorporate them into your life. Perhaps you've always been good at cooking and would like to try out new recipes but find yourself looping back to the same dishes time and again for ease. To break the cycle, offer to cook something new for friends or relatives and bring in a social element, or volunteer your time to teach others how to cook for themselves.

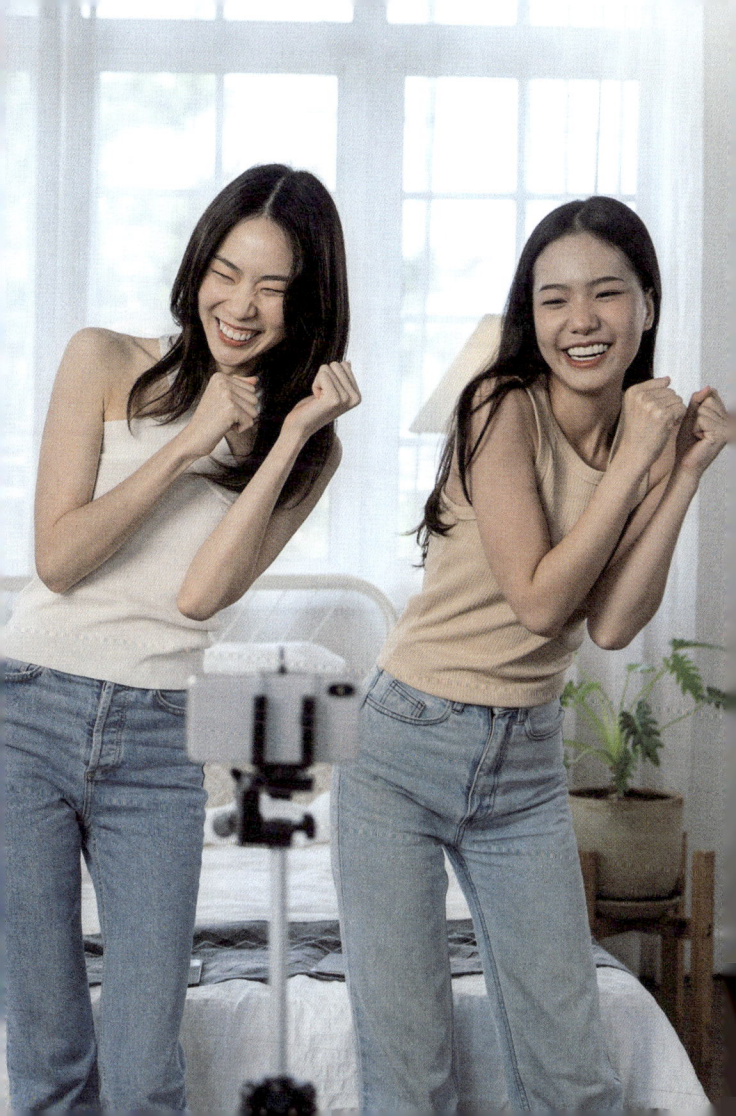

FOCUS ON YOUR STRENGTHS

It's important to remember that your ikigai is yours and no one else's. You seek it out, moulding it through your choices and integrating it into your life. Don't compare yourself to others along your journey or strive for someone else's idea of perfection.

Social media usually only tells one side of the story, and reality looks very different. Have a declutter of the accounts you follow or limit your time using social channels; there are apps to help you manage this if you find it difficult.

This would also be a good place to harness your affirmations (see page 80) and tell yourself, "There is no such thing as perfection: practice makes progress."

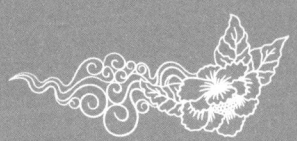

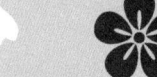

ACCEPT WHO
YOU ARE, AND
COMMIT TO
YOUR PURPOSE
WHOLEHEARTEDLY

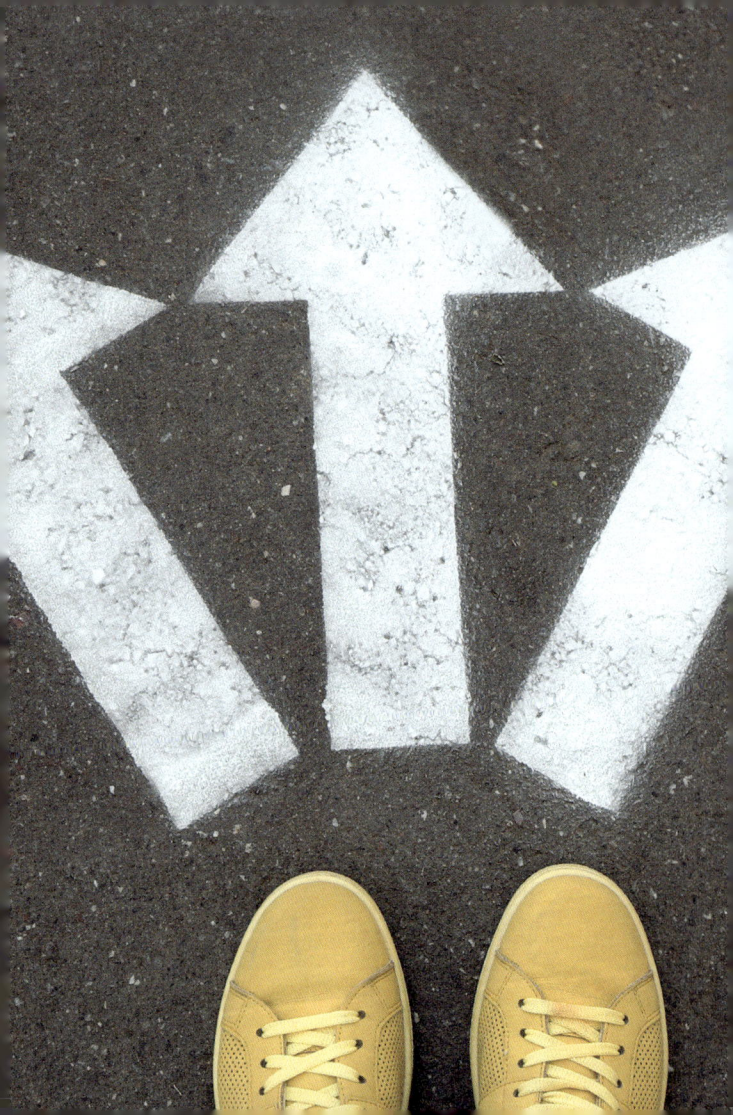

SHAPE YOUR CAREER

Balance is key to ikigai, so is your profession and the idea that finding satisfaction in different areas of your life will lead to happiness. This explains why the Japanese have no word for "retire", instead they encourage people to fulfil their professional ikigai by taking on new and different roles in later life.

Think of your career as an ever-evolving entity. Just because you trained in one area does not mean you can't move into another. According to The World Economic Forum's *Future of Jobs Report 2023*, due to the rapid pace of technological change we are embarking on an era where we will experience multiple career changes in our lifetime. Many roles that exist now will be phased out and workers will be required to update their skills in order to stay relevant. Harnessing these opportunities will help you stay ahead of the curve and find career fulfilment.

FIND YOUR
WORK–LIFE BALANCE

We often spend more time at work than we do with the people we love, so it's important to strive for contentment in this area of our lives to achieve the ultimate goal of a happy work–life balance. If your current job is getting you down, be mindful of whether it is the job itself or the conditions around it that is causing the issue. Look for solutions to any problems that have arisen and work with colleagues to resolve them.

When you feel you have exhausted all avenues, perhaps it's time to accept you need to look for something new. You could try asking yourself the questions on page 132 to help you identify the things that are most important to you at work. This will help you find your professional ikigai. You can also seek career advice about your transferable skills if you're not sure where to go next.

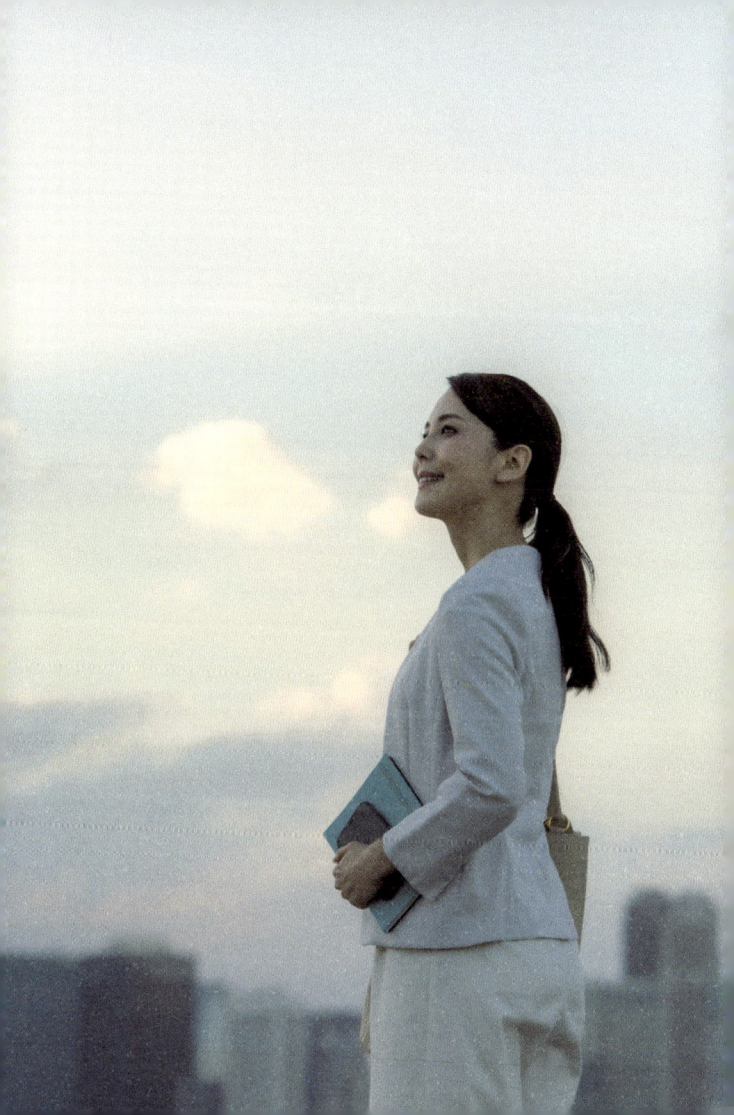

HAPPINESS AT WORK

Are you happy at work? Set aside some time to sit down and really ask yourself this question. Take a notepad and pen and write down the pros and cons of your current job. What are the hours like? What about the benefits? Do you get on with your co-workers? When you close your eyes and imagine what you might be doing for work in a year's time, are you still in the same role? What about two or even five years' time? Does the thought of still working with the same people and doing the same tasks leave you cold?

If it does, it might be time for a change – and there's no point in delaying the inevitable. Write yourself a plan and timeline detailing your next career move. Getting it all down on paper will help you take the steps to make it a reality.

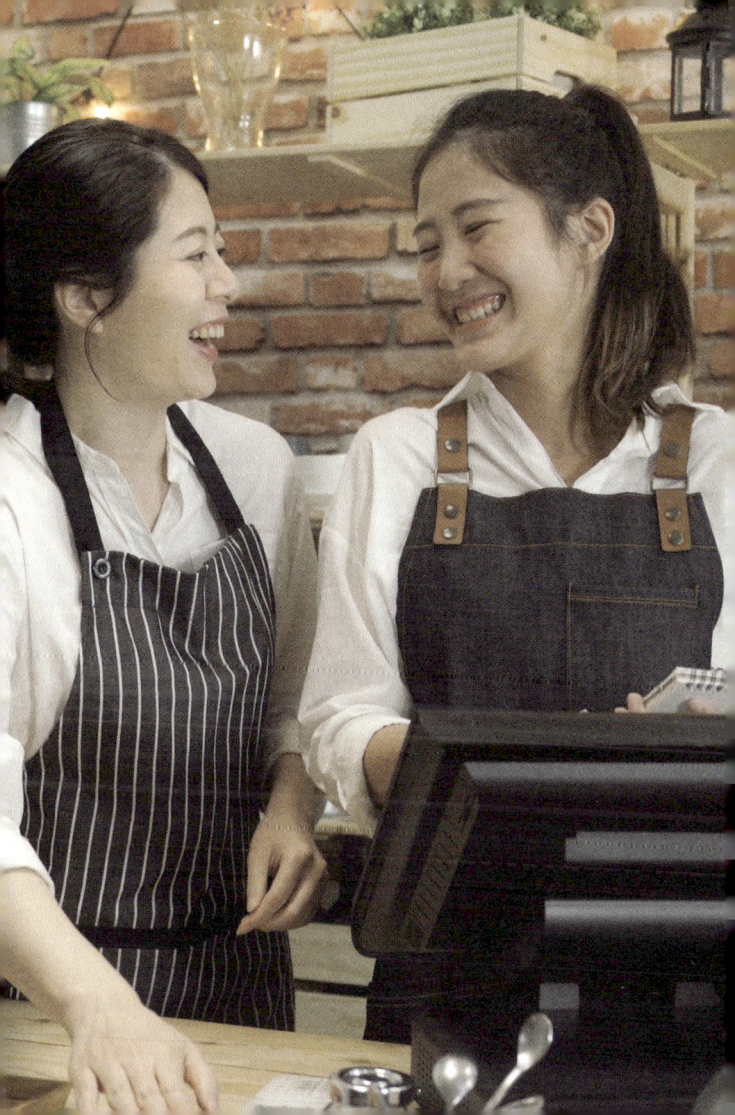

I quit my job
so I could focus on
my work instead.

TIM TAMASHIRO

TAKE BACK YOUR IKIGAI

There may well be times when you find yourself losing sight of your ikigai, as daily pressures take their toll and mounting priorities mean you must concentrate on others, leaving less time for yourself.

Try leaving subtle reminders for yourself around your home and on your devices to help you remember what you're working towards. These could be notes on your calendar, or simple sticky notes on a mirror or the fridge – places you look often. The notes could remind you to take a moment to reflect when you're going about your daily tasks. Also use calendar entries to block out larger chunks of time to dedicate to the things you enjoy, encouraging you to make space for these when it feels like there is none.

When you find you are focused intently on your ikigai and making progress on your journey, offer to help others find their way back to the path.

FILL YOUR LIFE WITH MEANING, HARMONY AND HAPPINESS

The most effective way
to do it is to do it.

AMELIA EARHART

CONCLUSION

While it's likely you were already aware of some of the things that made you happy, perhaps by reading this book you have been able to think about these things in terms of your sense of purpose and how they can fit into the bigger picture in your search for ikigai.

Remember, finding your ikigai is a journey – often a long one. It is also something that evolves over time as your life changes, so awareness of this and perseverance in your search are key. In these pages you have learned how to live with your ikigai once you have identified it – and discovered ways to maintain that sense of purpose throughout your life. Once you find your ikigai it is important to learn how to fine-tune it as your life changes in order to keep it with you always.

Using the learnings from this book to work on the four pillars – what you love, what the world needs, what you are good at and what you can be paid for – you will be able to search for deeper meaning in your daily life and combine your strengths to become more fulfilled. Bringing these key areas of your life in line with each other will require soul-searching, but will reveal what you are capable of and what you can achieve.

There may be times when you need to work harder than usual to hold on to your sense of being, but with the guidance in this book you will rediscover it in no time. To truly find ikigai is to take enjoyment from everything you choose to do. Help others who are struggling to realize their ikigai and you will feel even more fulfilled.

With ikigai on your side, you will harness the tools to live life in a more thoughtful way, to ultimately be healthier, happier and on the road to contentment. By embracing the Japanese wisdom of ikigai, you can change your life and find your purpose in the world.

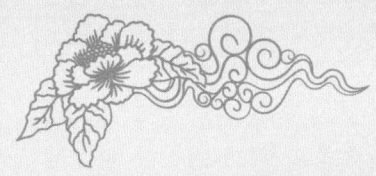

RESOURCES

APPS

Calm – Offering meditative tools to help with anxiety, sleep and relaxation.

Daylio – A "micro-diary" that allows you to track everything from fitness goals to moods.

Down Dog – Instructor-led yoga practice, featuring tips and personalized classes.

Headspace – A meditation app.

Ikigai DIY – A tool to set goals for all areas of your ikigai.

BOOKS

García, Héctor and Miralles, Francesc *Ikigai: The Japanese Secret to a Long and Happy Life* (2017, Hutchinson)

García, Héctor and Miralles, Francesc *The Ikigai Journey: A Practical Guide to Finding Happiness and Purpose the Japanese Way* (2020, Tuttle)

Longhurst, Erin Niimi *Japonisme* (2018, Harper Thorsens)

Tamashiro, Tim *How to Ikigai: Lessons for Finding Happiness and Living Your Life's Purpose* (2019, Mango)

PODCASTS

The High Performance Podcast (Episode from 7 April 2023: "Discovering Your Ikigai: Finding Purpose, Passion, and Fulfilment in Life with Hector García") – www.thehighperformancepodcast.com
Ikigai Tribe – www.ikigaitribe.com/podcasts

WEBSITES

Ikigai Tribe – www.ikigaitribe.com
Tim Tamashiro Ted Talk – www.ted.com/talks/tim_tamashiro_how_to_ikigai
Yoga with Adriene – www.yogawithadriene.com/free-yoga-videos

CREDITS

Cover and p.1 © R.Kido/Shutterstock.com; p.3 and throughout © ADELART/Shutterstock.com; pp.4–5 © Bossa Art/Shutterstock.com; p.6 and throughout © arifafrin/Shutterstock.com; p.9 © AsiaTravel/Shutterstock.com; pp.10–11 © Jo Panuwat D/Shutterstock.com; p.13 © K-Angle/Shutterstock.com; p.14 and throughout © burao_sato/Shutterstock.com; pp.16–17 © imtmphoto/Shutterstock.com; p.21 © Rapeepat Pornsipak/Shutterstock.com; pp.22–23 © Evgeny Atamanenko/Shutterstock.com; p.25 © rzoze19/Shutterstock.com; pp.28–29 © Sean Pavone/Shutterstock.com; pp.32–33 © Versta/Shutterstock.com; pp.38–39 © Rido/Shutterstock.com; p.41 © Kostikova Natalia/Shutterstock.com; pp.44–45 kapinon.stuio/Shutterstock.com; p.49 © PR Image Factory/Shutterstock.com; pp.50–51 © imtmphoto/Shutterstock.com; p.57 © Stock Rojo Verde y Azul/Shutterstock.com; pp.58–59 © metamorworks/Shutterstock.com; p.63 © zEdward_Indy/Shutterstock.com; pp.64–65 © SEALANDSKYPHOTO/Shutterstock.com; p.67 © Ground Picture/Shutterstock.com; pp.68–69 © 220 Selfmade studio/Shutterstock.com; p.71 © Kite_rin/Shutterstock.com; pp.72–73 © Antonio Guillem/Shutterstock.com; p.75 © kapinon.stuio/Shutterstock.com; pp.76–77 © photoK-jp/Shutterstock.com; p.81 © Jo Panuwat D/Shutterstock.com; pp.82–83 © metamorworks/Shutterstock.com; p.85 © PeopleImages.com -Yuri A/Shutterstock.com; pp.86–87 © Tanja Esser/Shutterstock.com; p.89 © Miljan Zivkovic/Shutterstock.com; pp.92–93 © PeopleImages.com – Yuri A/Shutterstock.com; p.95 © Cristina RasoBoluda/Shutterstock.com; pp.102–103 © Tammyiho/Shutterstock.com; p.105 © PeopleImages.com -Yuri A/Shutterstock.com; pp.106–107 © yamasan0708/Shutterstock.com; p.109 © Hananeko_Studio/Shutterstock.com; pp.110–111 © PeopleImages.com – Yuri A/Shutterstock.com; p.113 © SasinTipchai/Shutterstock.com; pp.116–117 © Bignai/Shutterstock.com; p.119 © addkm/Shutterstock.com; pp.122–123 © dodotone/Shutterstock.com; p.125 © paulaphoto/Shutterstock.com; pp.128–129 © New Africa/Shutterstock.com; p.131 © metamorworks/Shutterstock.com; pp.132–133 © PRPicturesProduction/Shutterstock.com; pp.138–139 © Pratchaya.Lee/Shutterstock.com

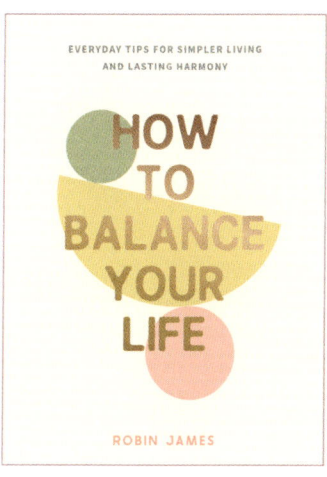

HOW TO BALANCE YOUR LIFE

Everyday Tips for Simpler Living and Lasting Harmony

Robin James

Hardback

ISBN:
978-1-83799-505-9

Find harmony in all aspects of your life with this beautiful guide to simple, balanced living

With practical tips on everything from managing day-to-day stress to finding a work–life balance, *How to Balance Your Life* is your go-to guide to discovering lasting peace and harmony. This inspirational book will help you find ways to boost your well-being and be more mindful of the wider world and your impact on it, while making sure there is always room for "me" time.

Have you enjoyed this book?
If so, why not write a review on
your favourite website?

If you're interested in finding out
more about our books, find us on
Facebook at Summersdale Publishers,
on Twitter/X at @Summersdale and
on Instagram, TikTok and Bluesky at
@summersdalebooks and get in touch.
We'd love to hear from you!

Thanks very much for buying this Summersdale book.

www.summersdale.com